THE COMPLETE DIABETES DIET AFTER 50

Unlocking Wellness through Nutrition and Lifestyle

ADOOH MARCEL

DEDICATION

This book is dedicated to God almighty and my entire family for their unwavering support, boundless encouragement, and profound love they have showered upon me throughout my life and in the course of writing this book. They are the beating heart of my existence, and I want the world to know just how profoundly I appreciate their presence in my journey. And I pray that the almighty God bless them all.

The Complete Diabetes Diet After 50

Copyright 2023 – Adooh Marcel

Table of Contents

INTRODUCTION

As we age, our bodies undergo various changes, and our health becomes a top priority. One of the health concerns that become more prevalent as we reach our 50s and beyond is diabetes. Diabetes is a chronic medical condition that affects how your body processes sugar, or glucose, and it can have a profound impact on your overall well-being. In this introductory guide, we will explore the complexities of diabetes, with a specific focus on diabetes after the age of 50.

For many individuals, the age of 50 marks a significant milestone in their lives. It can be a time of reflection, newfound goals, and a greater focus on health and well-being. Understanding diabetes in this context becomes crucial, as it is one of the most common chronic conditions to develop in older adults. Whether you have recently been diagnosed with diabetes, are concerned about your risk factors, or simply wish to learn more about this condition, this guide is here to provide you with the knowledge and insights you need.

In the following sections, we will delve into the following topics:

1. What is Diabetes? – We will provide a fundamental understanding of diabetes, its types, and how it affects the body's ability to regulate blood sugar levels.
2. Diabetes Risk Factors – Discover the factors that can increase your likelihood of developing diabetes, with a particular focus on those that become more relevant after the age of 50.
3. Symptoms and Diagnosis – Learn to recognize the signs and symptoms of diabetes and how it is diagnosed by healthcare professionals.
4. Managing Diabetes – Explore the various approaches to managing diabetes, including lifestyle changes, medication, and monitoring blood sugar levels.
5. Living with Diabetes – Gain insights into the daily challenges and considerations that come with living with diabetes, as well as

strategies for maintaining a fulfilling life while managing the condition.

6. Preventing and Reducing Diabetes Risk – Discover practical steps you can take to reduce your risk of developing diabetes or manage the condition effectively if you have been diagnosed.
7. Conclusion – Summarize the key takeaways and emphasize the importance of knowledge, early detection, and proactive management of diabetes after 50.

Throughout this guide, we will strive to provide you with valuable information, practical advice, and resources to help you navigate the complexities of diabetes in the later stages of life. By understanding diabetes after the age of 50 and taking appropriate steps, you can empower yourself to live a healthier, more fulfilling life.

THE IMPORTANCE OF DIET IN DIABETES MANAGEMENT

Diet plays a pivotal role in the management of diabetes, regardless of your age. However, as we age, the importance of maintaining a balanced and healthy diet becomes even more critical, especially for those who are 50 and older. Proper nutrition can help control blood sugar levels, prevent complications, and improve overall health. In this section, we will explore the significance of diet in diabetes management and provide some essential guidelines for individuals with diabetes, especially those in the later stages of life.

1. Blood Sugar Control: The carbohydrates you consume directly affect your blood sugar levels. Managing your carbohydrate intake is a fundamental aspect of controlling diabetes. Complex carbohydrates, such as whole grains, legumes, and vegetables, are generally better choices than simple sugars. Monitoring portion sizes and spreading carbohydrate intake throughout the day can help stabilize blood sugar levels.
2. Weight Management: Maintaining a healthy weight is crucial for diabetes management. Excess body weight can make it more challenging for your body to use insulin effectively. A balanced diet that supports weight control is essential, focusing on portion control and nutrient-dense foods.
3. Fiber-Rich Foods: Fiber helps regulate blood sugar levels and can also improve heart health. Incorporate foods like whole grains, fruits, vegetables, and legumes into your diet to increase fiber intake.
4. Healthy Fats: Opt for unsaturated fats, such as those found in nuts, seeds, avocados, and olive oil, while limiting saturated and trans fats. Healthy fats can help improve cholesterol levels and reduce the risk of heart disease, which is a common concern for people with diabetes.
5. Protein: Include lean sources of protein in your diet, such as poultry, fish, tofu, and legumes. Protein can help you feel full and provide a steady source of energy without causing rapid blood sugar spikes.

6. Meal Timing: Consistency in meal timing is crucial. Try to eat at regular intervals to help stabilize blood sugar levels and avoid large fluctuations. Skipping meals can lead to low blood sugar (hypoglycaemia) in individuals taking diabetes medications.

7. Sugar and Sugary Foods: Minimize your consumption of sugary foods and beverages. Sugary items can cause rapid spikes in blood sugar levels. Artificial sweeteners or sugar substitutes can be alternatives, but use them in moderation.

8. Monitoring and Adjusting: Regularly monitor your blood sugar levels as advised by your healthcare provider. This will help you understand how different foods affect your body and allow for necessary adjustments to your diet and medications.

9. Consult a Registered Dietitian: For personalized guidance, consult with a registered dietitian or nutritionist who specializes in diabetes care. They can help you create a customized meal plan that aligns with your specific needs and preferences.

10. Hydration: Staying well-hydrated is essential. Water is the best choice, and it can help regulate blood sugar levels.

In summary, diet is a cornerstone of diabetes management, especially as we age. Making informed food choices, maintaining a balanced diet, and working closely with healthcare professionals can greatly assist in controlling blood sugar levels and preventing diabetes-related complications. Remember that diabetes management should be tailored to your individual needs and preferences, and ongoing communication with your healthcare team is crucial for your overall well-being.

CHAPTER ONE
DIABETES BASICS

Diabetes is a chronic medical condition that affects how your body regulates blood sugar, or glucose. Glucose is a crucial source of energy for your cells and is obtained from the food you eat. To properly utilize glucose, your body relies on a hormone called insulin, which is produced by the pancreas. Diabetes disrupts the balance between glucose and insulin, resulting in elevated blood sugar levels, which can lead to various health complications.

HERE ARE SOME FUNDAMENTAL ASPECTS OF DIABETES:

TYPES OF DIABETES:
- **Type 1 Diabetes:** This is an autoimmune condition where the immune system mistakenly attacks and destroys the insulin-producing beta cells in the pancreas. People with type 1 diabetes need to take insulin injections or use an insulin pump to manage their blood sugar.
- **Type 2 Diabetes:** This is the most common form of diabetes and is often associated with lifestyle factors, genetics, and aging. In type 2 diabetes, the body becomes resistant to the effects of insulin, and the pancreas may not produce enough insulin to compensate.
- **Gestational Diabetes:** Some women develop diabetes during pregnancy, known as gestational diabetes. It typically resolves after childbirth, but it increases the risk of developing type 2 diabetes later in life.

SYMPTOMS OF DIABETES:
- Frequent urination
- Excessive thirst
- Unexplained weight loss
- Fatigue
- Blurred vision

- Slow-healing wounds
- Tingling or numbness in the extremities
- Increased hunger

DIAGNOSIS:

Diabetes is diagnosed through blood tests, including the fasting plasma glucose test, oral glucose tolerance test, and the HbA1c test, which measures average blood sugar levels over a few months.

MANAGEMENT:

- **Type 1 Diabetes:** Requires insulin therapy, blood sugar monitoring, and careful management of diet and exercise.
- **Type 2 Diabetes:** Managed through lifestyle changes, including diet and exercise, oral medications, and, in some cases, insulin therapy.
- **Gestational Diabetes:** Managed through dietary changes and, in some cases, medication. Regular monitoring and post-pregnancy follow-up are essential.

COMPLICATIONS:

Diabetes can lead to a range of complications, including:

- Heart disease and stroke
- Kidney disease
- Nerve damage (neuropathy)
- Eye problems (retinopathy)
- Foot problems, including diabetic foot ulcers
- Skin conditions
- Dental issues
- Cognitive decline

PREVENTION:

Lifestyle modifications, including a balanced diet, regular physical activity, weight management, and avoiding tobacco use, can help reduce the risk of type 2 diabetes.

MONITORING:

Regular monitoring of blood sugar levels is essential for diabetes management. This may involve daily self-monitoring at home or occasional lab tests.

SUPPORT:

Diabetes management often requires a multidisciplinary approach, involving healthcare professionals like endocrinologists, dietitians, and diabetes educators. Support from family and friends can also be invaluable.

Understanding the basics of diabetes is the first step in effectively managing and living with this condition. Whether you're newly diagnosed or providing support to someone with diabetes, education, regular healthcare check-ups, and a commitment to a healthy lifestyle are key components of long-term diabetes care.

PREVALENCE AND RISKS FOR PEOPLE OVER FIFTY (50)

Diabetes is a health concern that becomes more prevalent and poses specific risks for individuals over the age of 50. Understanding the prevalence and associated risks is crucial for effective management and prevention. Here's an overview of diabetes prevalence and associated risks in this age group:

1. **PREVALENCE**:
    - **Type 2 Diabetes**: Type 2 diabetes is more common in older adults, with a significant increase in prevalence after the age of 45. The risk continues to rise as individuals reach their 50s, 60s, and beyond.
    - **Gestational Diabetes**: While typically occurring in pregnant women, gestational diabetes can also affect older expectant mothers. The risk of gestational diabetes increases with age.
2. **RISKS**:
    - **Increased Insulin Resistance**: As people age, they often become more resistant to insulin, especially if they are sedentary and carry excess weight. This insulin resistance is a significant risk factor for type 2 diabetes.
    - **Sedentary Lifestyle**: Physical inactivity can lead to weight gain and reduced muscle mass, which further contributes to insulin resistance and the development of type 2 diabetes.

- **Obesity**: Excess body weight, especially around the abdomen, is a significant risk factor for type 2 diabetes. Older adults may find it more challenging to maintain a healthy weight.
- **Genetics**: Family history plays a role in diabetes risk. If there's a family history of diabetes, individuals over 50 should be particularly vigilant about lifestyle choices.
- **Poor Diet**: Unhealthy eating habits, such as a diet high in processed foods, sugary beverages, and excessive carbohydrates, can increase the risk of diabetes.
- **Hypertension**: High blood pressure is a common coexisting condition with diabetes and can further increase the risk of cardiovascular complications in older adults.
- **High Cholesterol**: Elevated cholesterol levels can also be a risk factor, contributing to the development of heart disease in individuals with diabetes.
- **Socioeconomic Factors**: Socioeconomic factors can impact access to healthcare, healthy food, and opportunities for physical activity, which can influence diabetes risk.

3. **COMPLICATIONS**: Older adults with diabetes are at a higher risk for various complications, including heart disease, stroke, kidney disease, nerve damage, vision problems, and foot problems. Additionally, managing diabetes becomes more complex as other age-related health issues may coexist.

4. **PREVENTION AND MANAGEMENT**: The management and prevention of diabetes in people over 50 often require a holistic approach. Lifestyle modifications, such as a balanced diet, regular physical activity, weight management, and blood sugar monitoring, are essential. Medications, including insulin or oral medications may be prescribed by healthcare providers. Regular healthcare check-ups to monitor blood sugar levels, blood pressure, cholesterol, and overall health are crucial for early intervention and risk reduction.

Understanding the prevalence and associated risks of diabetes in the 50-and-over age group underscores the importance of proactive measures for diabetes prevention and management. Lifestyle choices and ongoing healthcare support can help individuals in this age group lead healthier and more fulfilling lives, even in the presence of diabetes.

MANAGING DIABETES AT AN OLDER AGE

Diabetes management can present unique challenges as individuals age. Effective management is crucial for maintaining a good quality of life and preventing complications. Here are some key considerations and strategies for managing diabetes at an older age:

1. **Regular Monitoring**: Monitor your blood sugar levels regularly as advised by your healthcare provider. This helps you and your healthcare teams make informed decisions about your treatment plan.
2. **Medication Management**: If you are prescribed medication for diabetes, it's important to take it as directed. Older adults often have multiple medications, so it's essential to keep a medication schedule and consult your healthcare provider if you have concerns about interactions or side effects.
3. **Lifestyle Choices**:
     - **Diet**: Maintain a balanced diet with a focus on whole, nutrient-dense foods. Portion control is crucial. Consider consulting with a registered dietitian for personalized dietary guidance.
     - **Physical Activity**: Engage in regular physical activity suitable for your fitness level. Exercise can help improve insulin sensitivity, manage weight, and boost overall health.
     - **Weight Management**: Aim for a healthy weight. Even a modest weight loss can improve blood sugar control.
4. **Regular Medical Check-Ups**: Beyond diabetes, older adults may have other chronic conditions like hypertension and heart disease. Regular check-ups help manage these conditions and prevent complications.
5. **Foot Care**: Diabetes can affect blood flow to the feet and nerve function. Regularly inspect and care for your feet, and wear

comfortable shoes that fit well. Seek prompt medical attention for any foot problems.

6. **Eye Care**: Diabetes can lead to vision problems. Schedule regular eye exams to catch and treat issues early.

7. **Heart Health**: Manage cardiovascular risk factors, such as high blood pressure and cholesterol. A heart-healthy diet, regular exercise, and medications may be necessary.

8. **Dental Care**: Good oral hygiene is important, as gum disease can affect blood sugar control.

9. **Social Support**: Lean on friends and family for support. Discuss your diabetes management with them, and let them know how they can help in emergencies.

10. **Mental Health**: Managing diabetes can be emotionally challenging. It's important to address any stress, anxiety, or depression, which can affect blood sugar levels. Seek support from healthcare providers or mental health professionals when needed.

11. **Diabetes Education**: Consider attending diabetes education classes or working with a diabetes educator. They can provide valuable information, tips, and techniques for better self-management.

12. **Emergency Preparedness**: Have a plan in case of a hypoglycemic (low blood sugar) episode. Carry a source of glucose, like glucose tablets, and make sure family members know what to do in an emergency.

13. **Advance Care Planning**: As you age, it's important to have discussions about your healthcare wishes and preferences, especially related to diabetes management, with your family and healthcare providers.

14. **Medicare and Insurance Coverage**: Be aware of the coverage provided by your health insurance, especially Medicare, as it can play a significant role in accessing diabetes-related care and supplies.

15. **Medication Storage**: Ensure that your diabetes medications are stored properly and are not expired.

Managing diabetes at an older age involves a multidimensional approach that considers not only blood sugar control but also the prevention of complications and overall well-being. It's essential to work closely with your healthcare team to develop a personalized plan that addresses your specific needs and circumstances. With the right support and self-care, many older adults can effectively manage diabetes and enjoy a fulfilling life.

CHAPTER TWO
ASSESSING YOUR DIABETES

Assessing your diabetes is a critical step in understanding and managing the condition effectively. Regular self-assessment and medical check-ups help you monitor your blood sugar control and overall health. Here's a guide on how to assess your diabetes:

1. **Blood Sugar Monitoring**:
   - Regularly check your blood sugar levels using a blood glucose meter or continuous glucose monitoring system (CGM) as prescribed by your healthcare provider.
   - Keep a record of your blood sugar readings and patterns. Note any trends or consistent high or low readings.

2. **HbA1c Test**:
   - This blood test provides an average of your blood sugar levels over the past two to three months. It's typically done every 3 to 6 months.
   - The target HbA1c level varies by individual and is determined by your healthcare provider. It's usually around 7% for many people with diabetes.

3. **Regular Medical Check-Ups**:
   - Schedule regular check-ups with your healthcare provider. They will assess your overall health, perform physical exams, and review your blood sugar control.
   - Discuss any changes in your condition, medications, and any symptoms or concerns you may have.

4. **Foot Examination**:
   - As part of your regular check-ups, your healthcare provider should perform a foot examination to check for signs of neuropathy or circulation problems.
   - You can also conduct self-foot checks at home to look for any sores, wounds, or changes in your feet.

5. **Eye Exams**:
   - Regular eye exams are crucial to monitor for diabetes-related eye conditions like diabetic retinopathy.

- Follow your eye specialist's recommendations for the frequency of exams.

6. **Kidney Function**:
   - Periodic blood and urine tests can assess your kidney function, as diabetes can affect the kidneys.
   - Monitor for any signs of kidney problems and communicate them to your healthcare provider.

7. **Cholesterol and Blood Pressure**:
   - Keep an eye on your cholesterol levels and blood pressure, as people with diabetes are at higher risk for heart disease.
   - Maintain a heart-healthy diet and lifestyle to help control these risk factors.

8. **Weight Management**:
   - Regularly assess and manage your weight to ensure it remains within a healthy range. This can positively impact blood sugar control.

9. **Mental Health and Stress**:
   - Assess your mental well-being, as diabetes management can be stressful.
   - Seek support or counseling if you experience diabetes-related distress, anxiety, or depression.

10. **Medication and Insulin Management**:
    - Ensure you're taking your prescribed medications or insulin as directed and as scheduled.
    - Regularly review your medication plan with your healthcare provider, especially if there are changes in your lifestyle or health.

11. **Lifestyle Assessment**:
    - Evaluate your dietary choices, physical activity level, and any changes that could affect your diabetes management.
    - Consider consulting with a registered dietitian or diabetes educator for guidance.

12. **Emergency Preparedness**:
    - Assess your preparedness for hypoglycemic (low blood sugar) or hyperglycemic (high blood sugar) episodes. Ensure you have glucose sources on hand.

13. **Dental and Oral Health**:

- Maintain good oral hygiene and regular dental check-ups, as gum disease can affect blood sugar control.

14. **Advance Care Planning**:
    - Discuss your healthcare preferences, including those related to diabetes management, with your family and healthcare providers.

15. **Support System**:
    - Assess the support you have from family, friends, and healthcare professionals. A strong support system can make a significant difference in managing diabetes effectively.

Regularly assessing your diabetes and collaborating with your healthcare team are vital for effective management and overall well-being. The goal is to maintain stable blood sugar levels, prevent complications, and enjoy a fulfilling life while living with diabetes.

CHAPTER THREE
NUTRITION FUNDAMENTALS

Nutrition is a fundamental aspect of our lives that significantly impacts our health and well-being. It encompasses the intake of essential nutrients, the body's utilization of these nutrients, and the overall relationship between diet and health. Here are some key nutrition fundamentals:

1. **Essential Nutrients**: Nutrients are substances that the body needs for growth, development, energy production, and overall function. The six main classes of essential nutrients are:
   - Carbohydrates
   - Proteins
   - Fats
   - Vitamins
   - Minerals
   - Water
2. **Calories**: Calories are units of energy provided by the macronutrients (carbohydrates, proteins, and fats) in our food. The number of calories we consume should match our energy expenditure to maintain a healthy weight.
3. **Balanced Diet**: A balanced diet includes a variety of foods that provide all essential nutrients in the right proportions. This helps maintain health, support growth, and prevent nutritional deficiencies.
4. **Macronutrients**:
   - **Carbohydrates**: Provide energy and are found in foods like grains, fruits, vegetables, and legumes.
   - **Proteins**: Essential for building and repairing tissues and can be found in meat, poultry, fish, beans, and dairy products.
   - **Fats**: Important for energy, absorbing fat-soluble vitamins, and maintaining cell health. Sources include nuts, oils, and fatty fish.
5. **Micronutrients**:

- **Vitamins**: Organic compounds essential for various bodily functions. They are found in fruits, vegetables, and other foods.
- **Minerals**: Inorganic compounds required for several physiological processes. Common minerals include calcium, potassium, and iron.

6. **Hydration**: Water is vital for overall health. Staying well-hydrated is essential for digestion, temperature regulation, and maintaining bodily functions.
7. **Portion Control**: Eating appropriate portion sizes helps manage calorie intake and prevents overeating.
8. **Whole Foods**: Whole, unprocessed foods are generally healthier than heavily processed options. They are typically higher in nutrients and fiber.
9. **Dietary Guidelines**: Most countries have dietary guidelines or recommendations that provide information on what constitutes a healthy diet. These guidelines can help individuals make informed choices.
10. **Nutrition Labels**: Reading nutrition labels on packaged foods can help you understand the nutritional content and make healthier choices.
11. **Personalization**: Nutritional needs vary from person to person based on factors like age, sex, activity level, and health conditions. It's important to tailor your diet to your specific requirements.
12. **Special Diets**: Some people may have dietary restrictions or preferences, such as vegetarianism, veganism, gluten-free diets, or specific medical diets. It's important to ensure that these diets still provide all essential nutrients.
13. **Moderation**: Enjoying occasional treats is fine, but moderation is key. Overconsumption of unhealthy foods can lead to health problems.
14. **Allergies and Intolerances**: Some individuals have food allergies or intolerances that require them to avoid specific foods. It's essential to identify and manage these conditions.
15. **Nutrition and Health**: A well-balanced diet plays a significant role in preventing chronic diseases such as heart disease, diabetes, and

obesity. Proper nutrition also supports immune function and overall well-being.

16. **Consult a Professional**: If you have specific nutritional concerns, health conditions, or dietary goals, consider consulting a registered dietitian or nutritionist. They can provide personalized guidance.

Understanding these nutrition fundamentals and applying them to your daily life can help you make informed food choices and prioritize your health and well-being. Good nutrition is the foundation for a healthy and fulfilling life.

CHAPTER FOUR
BUILDING A HEALTHY DIABETES DIET

If you have diabetes, managing your diet is crucial to controlling your blood sugar levels and preventing complications. Here are some steps to help you build a healthy diabetes diet:

1. **Consult a Registered Dietitian**: A registered dietitian with expertise in diabetes can help you create a personalized meal plan that suits your specific needs and preferences.
2. **Balanced Carbohydrates**: Carbohydrates significantly impact blood sugar levels. Focus on complex carbohydrates, such as whole grains, legumes, and non-starchy vegetables. These foods have a lower impact on blood sugar than simple carbohydrates like sugary snacks and white bread.
3. **Portion Control**: Managing portion sizes is essential. Use measuring cups or a food scale to control portions, and be mindful of your carbohydrate intake.
4. **Fiber-Rich Foods**: Include high-fiber foods like whole grains, fruits, vegetables, and legumes in your diet. Fiber can help stabilize blood sugar levels and improve digestive health.
5. **Lean Proteins**: Opt for lean sources of protein like poultry, fish, tofu, and legumes. Protein can help control hunger and stabilize blood sugar levels.
6. **Healthy Fats**: Choose unsaturated fats, such as those found in nuts, seeds, avocados, and olive oil. Limit saturated and trans fats, which can raise cholesterol levels and increase the risk of heart disease.
7. **Limit Sugary Foods**: Minimize your consumption of sugary foods and beverages. Artificial sweeteners or sugar substitutes can be alternatives, but use them in moderation.
8. **Regular Meal Timing**: Consistency in meal timing is crucial. Eating at regular intervals can help stabilize blood sugar levels and prevent large fluctuations.

9. **Monitor Blood Sugar Levels**: Regularly check your blood sugar levels as advised by your healthcare provider. This helps you understand how different foods affect your body and allows for necessary adjustments to your diet and medications.
10. **Hydration**: Stay well-hydrated with water, as it helps regulate blood sugar levels and overall health.
11. **Limit Processed Foods**: Processed foods are often high in sodium, unhealthy fats, and added sugars. Minimize your consumption of these foods, as they can negatively affect your health.
12. **Meal Planning**: Plan your meals and snacks in advance to ensure you're making healthy choices throughout the day. Having a structured meal plan can also help with portion control.
13. **Glycemic Index**: Consider the glycemic index (GI) of foods. Foods with a lower GI are digested more slowly and have a smaller impact on blood sugar levels. However, remember that the overall composition of the meal matters more than the GI of individual foods.
14. **Exercise**: Regular physical activity is an important part of diabetes management. It helps your body use insulin more effectively and can help control blood sugar levels.
15. **Alcohol**: If you consume alcohol, do so in moderation and with food. Alcohol can affect blood sugar levels and should be consumed with caution.
16. **Blood Pressure and Cholesterol**: Manage your blood pressure and cholesterol levels, as people with diabetes are at a higher risk of heart disease. A heart-healthy diet can help with this.
17. **Educate Yourself**: Continuously educate yourself about diabetes, nutrition, and the latest research and recommendations. Knowledge is empowering when it comes to managing your health.

Building a healthy diabetes diet is not a one-size-fits-all approach. It requires personalized adjustments based on your specific needs and how your body responds to different foods. Regular communication with your healthcare team and a proactive approach to managing your diet can significantly enhance your quality of life while living with diabetes.

CREATING A BALANCED PLATE

Balancing your plate with the right mix of nutrients is essential for maintaining stable blood sugar levels, managing your weight, and promoting overall health, especially if you have diabetes. The "plate method" is a simple and effective way to achieve a balanced diet. Here's how to create a balanced plate:

1. **Divide Your Plate**:
   - **Half Your Plate - Non-Starchy Vegetables**: Fill half of your plate with non-starchy vegetables like leafy greens, broccoli, cauliflower, bell peppers, and asparagus. These are low in calories and carbohydrates and provide essential vitamins and minerals.
   - **Quarter of Your Plate - Lean Protein**: Use a quarter of your plate for lean protein sources. Examples include skinless poultry, fish, tofu, beans, and lentils. Protein helps control hunger and maintain muscle mass.
   - **Quarter of Your Plate - Carbohydrates**: The remaining quarter of your plate should contain carbohydrates. Choose complex carbohydrates like whole grains (brown rice, quinoa, and whole wheat pasta), sweet potatoes, or legumes. These carbohydrates have a slower impact on blood sugar.
2. **Healthy Fats**:
   - Incorporate healthy fats into your meals, but use them in moderation. These can include a small portion of avocado, a drizzle of olive oil on your salad, or a handful of nuts.
3. **Watch Your Portions**:
   - Be mindful of portion sizes. Use measuring cups or a food scale if necessary, especially when it comes to carbohydrates.
4. **Fiber**:
   - Include high-fiber foods like whole grains, fruits, and vegetables in your meal. Fiber aids digestion and helps regulate blood sugar levels.
5. **Hydration**:
   - Drink water with your meals, as it aids digestion and helps maintain proper hydration.

6. **Variety**:
   - Aim for variety in your food choices to ensure you get a wide range of nutrients. Different colors of fruits and vegetables, for instance, provide different vitamins and minerals.
7. **Control Sugary Foods and Beverages**:
   - Limit sugary foods and beverages. If you choose to consume them, do so in moderation and with an awareness of their impact on your blood sugar.
8. **Consistency**:
   - Try to eat meals and snacks at regular intervals. Consistency in your meal schedule can help stabilize blood sugar levels.
9. **Avoid Processed Foods**:
   - Processed and highly refined foods often contain added sugars and unhealthy fats. Minimize their consumption and opt for whole, unprocessed foods.
10. **Monitor Blood Sugar**:
    - Regularly monitor your blood sugar levels as advised by your healthcare provider. This will help you understand how your meal choices affect your body.
11. **Consult a Registered Dietitian**:
    - If you're unsure about how to create a balanced plate or have specific dietary concerns, consider consulting a registered dietitian or diabetes educator who can provide personalized guidance.

Remember that individual dietary needs may vary, and it's important to tailor your plate to your specific health goals and blood sugar responses. The balanced plate method is a versatile approach that can be adapted to meet your nutritional needs while supporting your diabetes management and overall well-being.

THE ROLE OF FIBER IN A HEALTHY DIET

Fiber is an essential component of a healthy diet and plays a significant role in supporting overall health, including its importance in managing diabetes. Here are the key roles of fiber:

1. **Blood Sugar Control**:

- Soluble fiber, found in foods like oats, legumes, and some fruits, can help stabilize blood sugar levels. It does this by slowing the absorption of sugar, which can prevent rapid spikes in blood glucose after meals.

2. **Weight Management**:
   - Fiber-rich foods tend to be filling and can help control appetite, which is important for weight management. Maintaining a healthy weight is an integral part of diabetes management.

3. **Digestive Health**:
   - Insoluble fiber, found in foods like whole grains and vegetables, adds bulk to stool and helps prevent constipation. A healthy digestive system is important for overall well-being.

4. **Heart Health**:
   - Fiber can help reduce the risk of heart disease by lowering cholesterol levels. Soluble fiber binds to cholesterol and helps remove it from the body.

5. **Gut Health**:
   - Fiber acts as prebiotic, providing nourishment for beneficial gut bacteria. A healthy gut microbiome is linked to numerous health benefits, including better digestion and a strengthened immune system.

6. **Reduced Risk of Type 2 Diabetes**:
   - A diet high in fiber may reduce the risk of developing type 2 diabetes, as it can improve insulin sensitivity and lower the risk of insulin resistance.

7. **Prevention of Colon Cancer**:
   - High-fiber diets have been associated with a reduced risk of colon cancer. Fiber helps keep the digestive tract healthy and may reduce exposure to harmful substances in the colon.

8. **Lowering Blood Pressure**:
   - Some studies suggest that dietary fiber, particularly from whole grains, may help lower blood pressure. Controlling blood pressure is important for individuals with diabetes, as they are at a higher risk of heart disease.

To incorporate more fiber into your diet:

- Choose whole grains over refined grains, such as brown rice instead of white rice or whole wheat bread instead of white bread.
- Increase your intake of fruits and vegetables. The skin of fruits and vegetables often contains fiber, so leaving it on when possible is beneficial.
- Include legumes like lentils, beans, and peas in your meals.
- Snack on nuts and seeds, which are good sources of fiber.
- Gradually increase your fiber intake to prevent digestive discomfort, and drink plenty of water to help fiber move through your digestive system smoothly.

When adding more fiber to your diet, it's important to monitor your blood sugar levels and work with your healthcare provider or registered dietitian to ensure your dietary choices align with your diabetes management plan.

THE IMPORTANCE OF WHOLE FOODS

Whole foods are essential components of a healthy diet, and their consumption is particularly valuable in managing diabetes and promoting overall well-being. Here's why whole foods are important:

1. **Nutrient Density**:
   - Whole foods are rich in essential nutrients, including vitamins, minerals, antioxidants, and dietary fiber. These nutrients are vital for maintaining good health and preventing chronic diseases, including diabetes.
2. **Balanced Nutrition**:
   - Whole foods provide a balanced combination of macronutrients (carbohydrates, proteins, and fats) and micronutrients (vitamins and minerals). This balance helps support overall health and stable blood sugar levels.
3. **Fiber Content**:

- Whole foods, such as whole grains, fruits, vegetables, and legumes, are high in dietary fiber. Fiber aids in digestion, helps control blood sugar levels, and promotes a feeling of fullness, which can assist with weight management.

4. **Lower Glycemic Index**:
   - Many whole foods have a lower glycemic index (GI) compared to processed and refined foods. Lower-GI foods cause a slower, more gradual increase in blood sugar levels, making them suitable choices for individuals with diabetes.

5. **Minimized Processing**:
   - Whole foods are minimally processed or not processed at all. This means they retain their natural state and are free from added sugars, unhealthy fats, and artificial additives.

6. **Digestive Health**:
   - The fiber in whole foods supports a healthy digestive system by preventing constipation, promoting regular bowel movements, and supporting the growth of beneficial gut bacteria.

7. **Weight Management**:
   - Whole foods are typically less calorie-dense than processed foods. Incorporating them into your diet can help control calorie intake and support weight management.

8. **Reduced Risk of Chronic Diseases**:
   - A diet rich in whole foods has been linked to a lower risk of chronic diseases, including heart disease, stroke, cancer, and diabetes.

9. **Satiety and Appetite Control**:
   - Whole foods tend to be more filling, which can help control hunger and prevent overeating. This is valuable for individuals with diabetes who need to manage their food intake.

10. **Heart Health**:
    - Many whole foods, such as fruits, vegetables, and whole grains, are heart-healthy and can help lower the risk of heart disease. People with diabetes are at a higher risk of heart-related complications.

11. **Diversity of Nutrients**:

- Consuming a variety of whole foods ensures that you obtain a wide range of essential nutrients, each with its unique health benefits.

EXAMPLES OF WHOLE FOODS INCLUDE:

- Whole grains (e.g., brown rice, quinoa, oats)
- Fresh fruits and vegetables
- Legumes (e.g., beans, lentils)
- Lean proteins (e.g., chicken, fish, tofu)
- Nuts and seeds
- Unprocessed dairy products (e.g., plain yogurt)

Incorporating whole foods into your diet is a cornerstone of a healthy eating plan for diabetes. When planning meals, focus on these nutritious options to optimize blood sugar control, support overall health, and reduce the risk of diabetes-related complications.

CHAPTER FIVE
MEAL PLANNING FOR DIABETES MANAGEMENT

Meal planning is a crucial aspect of managing diabetes as it helps you control blood sugar levels, maintain a healthy weight, and support overall well-being. Here's a step-by-step guide to effective meal planning for diabetes:

1. **Consult a Registered Dietitian**: If you're unsure where to start, consider consulting a registered dietitian who specializes in diabetes care. They can help you create a personalized meal plan tailored to your specific needs, preferences, and lifestyle.
2. **Understanding Carbohydrates**:
    - Carbohydrates have the most significant impact on blood sugar levels. Learn to identify sources of carbohydrates in your diet, such as grains, fruits, starchy vegetables, legumes, and dairy products.
3. **Portion Control**:
    - Be mindful of portion sizes to help manage calorie intake and blood sugar levels. Use measuring cups, a food scale, or visual cues to estimate appropriate portions.
4. **Balanced Plates**:
    - Follow the balanced plate method, where you fill half your plate with non-starchy vegetables, a quarter with lean protein, and a quarter with complex carbohydrates (e.g., whole grains).
5. **Fiber-Rich Foods**:
    - Include high-fiber foods like whole grains, vegetables, and legumes to support digestion and blood sugar control.
6. **Healthy Fats**:
    - Incorporate sources of healthy fats, such as avocados, olive oil, nuts, and seeds, in moderation to support heart health.
7. **Regular Meal Timing**:

- Aim to eat meals and snacks at regular intervals. Consistency in meal timing can help stabilize blood sugar levels.

8. **Glycemic Index (GI)**:
   - Be aware of the glycemic index of foods. Lower-GI foods are digested more slowly and have a smaller impact on blood sugar levels. However, consider the overall composition of your meals.

9. **Snacking**:
   - Plan healthy snacks if needed. Snacks can help prevent extreme blood sugar fluctuations between meals.

10. **Hydration**:
    - Stay well-hydrated with water, as it aids digestion and helps maintain proper hydration. Limit sugary drinks.

11. **Meal Prepping**:
    - Prepare meals and snacks in advance to ensure you have nutritious options readily available, especially during busy days.

12. **Monitoring Blood Sugar**:
    - Regularly monitor your blood sugar levels as recommended by your healthcare provider. This will help you understand how different foods affect your body.

13. **Tracking and Record-Keeping**:
    - Keep a food diary or use a mobile app to track your food intake and blood sugar levels. This can help identify patterns and make necessary adjustments to your meal plan.

14. **Consulting Your Healthcare Team**:
    - Share your meal plan and blood sugar records with your healthcare team during regular check-ups. They can provide guidance and adjust your treatment plan if necessary.

15. **Lifestyle Considerations**:
    - Take into account your physical activity level, stress, and any medications or insulin you may be taking when planning meals. All these factors can impact blood sugar levels.

16. **Enjoying Food**:
    - Make sure your meal plan is enjoyable and sustainable. You don't have to give up your favorite foods entirely but may need to adjust portion sizes and frequency.

17. **Educate Yourself**: Continuously educate yourself about diabetes, nutrition, and the latest research and recommendations. Knowledge is empowering when it comes to managing your health.

Effective meal planning is a dynamic process that involves adapting to your specific needs and goals. Regular communication with your healthcare team and a proactive approach to managing your diet can significantly enhance your quality of life while living with diabetes.

BREAKFAST IDEAS

CERTAINLY, HERE ARE SOME MORE BREAKFAST IDEAS:

1   **Overnight Oats**:
    - Combine rolled oats with unsweetened almond milk or low-fat yogurt, and add your favorite toppings such as fresh fruit, nuts, and a drizzle of honey or a sugar-free sweetener. Let it sit in the fridge overnight for a quick and nutritious breakfast.

2   **Nut Butter and Banana Roll-Up**:
    - Spread almond or peanut butter on a whole-grain tortilla, add banana slices, and roll it up for a portable and satisfying breakfast.

3   **Veggie Breakfast Wrap**:
    - Fill a whole-grain tortilla with scrambled eggs, sautéed spinach, tomatoes, and a sprinkle of feta cheese. Roll it up for a flavorful breakfast wrap.

4   **Quinoa Breakfast Bowl**:
    - Cook quinoa and top it with fresh berries, a dollop of Greek yogurt, and a drizzle of honey for a protein-rich and nutrient-packed breakfast.

5   **Egg and Cheese Breakfast Sandwich**:
    - Place scrambled eggs and a slice of low-fat cheese between whole-grain English muffins or bread for a satisfying breakfast sandwich.

6   **Leftover Dinner for Breakfast**:

- Leftovers from last night's dinner, such as grilled chicken, roasted vegetables, or stir-fried tofu, can be a quick and convenient breakfast option.

7 **Cottage Cheese and Fruit Salad**:
- Combine low-fat cottage cheese with a variety of fresh fruits like pineapple, melon, and grapes for a protein-packed and refreshing breakfast.

8 **Mini Frittatas**:
- Prepare mini frittatas using muffin tins. Mix eggs with diced vegetables and a small amount of cheese, pour the mixture into muffin cups, and bake until set. You can make these ahead for a grab-and-go breakfast.

9 **Smoked Salmon and Whole Grain Bagel**:
- Enjoy a whole-grain bagel with a spread of light cream cheese, smoked salmon, and capers for a nutritious and satisfying breakfast.

10 **Cherry Tomatoes and Mozzarella**:
- Pair cherry tomatoes with mozzarella cheese, fresh basil leaves, and a drizzle of balsamic vinegar for a simple and flavorful breakfast.

11 **High-Fiber Cereal with Berries**:
- Choose a high-fiber, low-sugar cereal and top it with a generous serving of fresh berries. Add unsweetened almond milk for extra creaminess.

12 **Baked Beans on Whole Grain Toast**:
- Heat up a serving of low-sugar baked beans and serve them on whole grain toast for a hearty and protein-rich breakfast.

13 **Mushroom and Spinach Breakfast Quesadilla**:
- Sauté mushrooms, spinach, and a sprinkle of cheese in a whole-grain tortilla for a savory breakfast option.

14 **Protein-Packed Smoothie Bowl**:
- Blend a smoothie using unsweetened almond milk, protein powder, spinach, and your favorite fruits. Pour it into a bowl and top with granola, nuts, and seeds for added texture.

These breakfast ideas offer a variety of options to suit your taste preferences and dietary requirements while supporting your diabetes management. Always monitor your blood sugar levels and consult with a healthcare provider or registered dietitian for personalized guidance.

LUNCH AND DINNER RECIPES FOR DIABETES MANAGEMENT

Here are some balanced lunch and dinner recipes suitable for individuals with diabetes. These recipes incorporate whole foods and focus on providing a good balance of carbohydrates, protein, and healthy fats:

LUNCH RECIPES:

1. **Grilled Chicken and Quinoa Salad**:
   - Grill chicken breast and serve it over a bed of cooked quinoa. Add mixed greens, cherry tomatoes, cucumber, and a vinaigrette dressing. This protein-packed salad is low in carbohydrates.
2. **Veggie Wrap**:
   - Fill a whole-grain tortilla with hummus, mixed greens, sliced bell peppers, cucumber, and shredded carrots. Roll it up for a quick and fiber-rich lunch.
3. **Tuna Salad**:
   - Mix canned tuna with Greek yogurt, diced celery, and a dash of mustard. Serve the tuna salad over a bed of lettuce or on whole-grain bread for a protein-rich meal.
4. **Egg Salad Lettuce Wraps**:
   - Make egg salad by mixing hard-boiled eggs, Greek yogurt, and Dijon mustard. Serve the egg salad in large lettuce leaves for a low-carb alternative to traditional sandwiches.
5. **Quinoa and Black Bean Bowl**:
   - Combine cooked quinoa, black beans, diced tomatoes, corn, and avocado. Top with a squeeze of lime juice for a flavorful and fiber-rich lunch.

DINNER RECIPES:

1. **Grilled Salmon with Asparagus and Brown Rice:**
   - Grill salmon with a drizzle of olive oil and season with herbs and spices. Serve it with steamed asparagus and brown rice for a balanced dinner.
2. **Chicken Stir-Fry:**
   - Stir-fry lean chicken breast with a mix of colorful vegetables (bell peppers, broccoli, snap peas) and a low-sodium stir-fry sauce. Serve it over brown rice or cauliflower rice.
3. **Vegetarian Chili:**
   - Make a hearty chili with a variety of beans, tomatoes, and vegetables. Season with chili spices and enjoy a fiber-rich and satisfying dinner.
4. **Baked Sweet Potato and Chickpea Curry:**
   - Roast sweet potato and chickpeas with a flavorful curry sauce. Serve over brown rice for a plant-based, protein-rich dinner.
5. **Grilled Veggie and Quinoa Stuffed Peppers:**
   - Stuff bell peppers with a mixture of grilled vegetables, cooked quinoa, and a touch of feta cheese. Bake until tender for a nutritious and colorful meal.
6. **Pork Tenderloin with Roasted Brussels Sprouts:**
   - Roast pork tenderloin with a balsamic glaze and serve with roasted Brussels sprouts. This dish is low in carbohydrates and rich in protein.
7. **Mushroom and Spinach Stuffed Chicken Breast:**
   - Stuff chicken breast with sautéed mushrooms and spinach. Bake until the chicken is cooked through, and serve it with a side of steamed broccoli.
8. **Zucchini Noodles with Pesto and Cherry Tomatoes:**
   - Spiralize zucchini into noodles and toss them with homemade pesto and cherry tomatoes. This low-carb pasta alternative is delicious and easy to prepare.

These lunch and dinner recipes offer a variety of options to suit your dietary preferences and diabetes management goals. Remember to monitor your blood sugar levels and consult with a healthcare provider or registered dietitian for personalized guidance on meal planning.

HEALTHY SNACK OPTIONS FOR DIABETES MANAGEMENT

Choosing the right snacks is crucial for managing blood sugar levels and preventing overeating. Here are some healthy snack options for individuals with diabetes:

1. **Raw Veggies with Hummus**:
   - Enjoy baby carrots, cucumber slices, cherry tomatoes, and bell pepper strips with a side of hummus for a crunchy and satisfying snack.
2. **Greek Yogurt with Berries**:
   - Opt for low-fat or non-fat Greek yogurt and top it with fresh berries for a protein-rich and antioxidant-packed snack.
3. **Apple Slices with Peanut Butter**:
   - Slice apples and dip them in natural peanut butter or almond butter. The combination of fiber and healthy fats will help keep you full.
4. **Nuts and Seeds**:
   - A small handful of mixed nuts and seeds, such as almonds, walnuts, and chia seeds, can provide healthy fats and protein for a filling snack.
5. **Cottage Cheese with Pineapple**:
   - Combine low-fat cottage cheese with pineapple chunks for a protein-packed and sweet treat.
6. **Hard-Boiled Eggs**:
   - Hard-boiled eggs are an excellent source of protein and make for a convenient and portable snack.
7. **String Cheese**:
   - Low-fat string cheese is a convenient and portion-controlled snack that provides protein and calcium.
8. **Sliced Avocado on Whole-Grain Crackers**:
   - Spread sliced avocado on whole-grain crackers for a satisfying snack that offers healthy fats and fiber.

9. **Cherry Tomatoes and Mozzarella**:
   - Pair cherry tomatoes with mozzarella cheese for a flavorful and easy-to-assemble snack.
10. **Berries and Cottage Cheese**:
    - Mix fresh berries with low-fat cottage cheese to enjoy a protein-rich and antioxidant-filled snack.
11. **Homemade Popcorn**:
    - Pop your own popcorn using plain kernels and season with a small amount of salt or your favorite spices for a whole-grain and low-calorie snack.
12. **Edamame**:
    - Steamed edamame (young soybeans) is a protein-rich and fiber-packed snack that you can enjoy hot or cold.
13. **Roasted Chickpeas**:
    - Roast chickpeas with your choice of spices for a crunchy and protein-packed snack.
14. **Yogurt Parfait**:
    - Layer non-fat yogurt with fresh fruit and a small sprinkle of granola or crushed nuts for a balanced and satisfying snack.
15. **Homemade Vegetable Chips**:
    - Make your own vegetable chips by thinly slicing sweet potatoes, zucchini, or kale, and baking them until crispy.
16. **Chia Pudding**:
    - Make chia pudding by mixing chia seeds with unsweetened almond milk, a dash of vanilla extract, and a sugar-free sweetener. Let it sit in the fridge for a creamy and nutritious snack.

Remember to monitor your blood sugar levels and consult with a healthcare provider or registered dietitian for personalized guidance on selecting snacks that align with your diabetes management plan.

MANAGING SPECIAL OCCASIONS WITH DIABETES

Special occasions, such as holidays, birthdays, and social gatherings, often involve a wide variety of foods and may pose challenges for individuals with diabetes. However, with careful planning and smart choices, you can enjoy these occasions while effectively managing your blood sugar levels. Here are some tips for managing special occasions with diabetes:

1. **Plan Ahead**:
   - Knowing what foods will be available allows you to plan your meals and snacks for the day. If possible, ask the host about the menu or offer to bring a diabetes-friendly dish.
2. **Monitor Your Blood Sugar**:
   - Regularly check your blood sugar levels before, during, and after the event to track how different foods affect you and make any necessary adjustments.
3. **Portion Control**:
   - Be mindful of portion sizes. Take small servings of higher-carb foods and balance them with non-starchy vegetables and lean proteins.
4. **Choose Wisely**:
   - Opt for foods that are lower in carbohydrates and sugar. Fill your plate with lean proteins, salads, and non-starchy vegetables.
5. **Limit Sugary Drinks**:
   - Avoid or limit sugary beverages and alcoholic drinks. Opt for water, unsweetened tea, or diet versions if available.
6. **Snack Beforehand**:
   - Have a healthy snack before attending the event to curb your appetite and prevent overindulging on less healthy options.
7. **Stay Active**:
   - Engage in physical activity before or after the event to help manage blood sugar levels.
8. **Watch the Desserts**:
   - If you want to indulge in dessert, choose smaller portions and consider sharing with a friend. Alternatively, look for options that are lower in sugar, such as fresh fruit.
9. **Stay Hydrated**:
   - Drink water throughout the event to stay hydrated, which can help control blood sugar levels.
10. **Inform Others**:

- Let your friends and family know about your dietary needs and preferences. They may be more understanding and supportive when it comes to food choices.

11. **Moderation is Key**:
    - It's okay to enjoy a treat occasionally, but be mindful of portion sizes and avoid overindulging.

12. **Carry Snacks**:
    - If you're unsure about the available food options, carry some diabetes-friendly snacks in your bag. This can help you avoid unhealthy choices in case there are limited options for you.

13. **Meal Timing**:
    - If the event disrupts your usual meal schedule, discuss with your healthcare provider about adjusting your medications or insulin as needed.

14. **Stress Management**:
    - High-stress levels can affect blood sugar. Practice stress-reduction techniques like deep breathing, meditation, or yoga to help manage your emotions during special occasions.

15. **Support System**:
    - Share your concerns and strategies with a trusted friend or family member who can provide support and encouragement.

16. **Enjoy the Company**:
    - Special occasions are about more than just the food. Focus on socializing, making memories, and enjoying the company of loved ones.

Remember that managing diabetes during special occasions is about finding a balance that works for you. Your healthcare provider and registered dietitian can provide personalized guidance and help you make informed decisions about your dietary choices to ensure you can enjoy these events while keeping your blood sugar in check.

CHAPTER SIX
SWEETENERS AND DIABETES

Artificial sweeteners, sugar substitutes, and natural sweeteners are commonly used by individuals with diabetes to add sweetness to their foods and beverages without causing a rapid spike in blood sugar. Here's an overview of different sweeteners and their implications for diabetes management:

1. **Artificial Sweeteners**:
   - Artificial sweeteners like aspartame (e.g., Equal, NutraSweet), saccharin (e.g., Sweet'N Low), sucralose (e.g., Splenda), and acesulfame potassium (e.g., Sunett) are sugar-free and have zero or very few calories.
   - They do not significantly affect blood sugar levels and can be used as sugar substitutes in a variety of foods and drinks.
   - Artificial sweeteners are considered safe when consumed within acceptable daily intake levels established by regulatory agencies, such as the U.S. Food and Drug Administration (FDA).
2. **Sugar Alcohols (Polyols)**:
   - Sugar alcohols like xylitol, erythritol, and sorbitol are commonly used as sugar substitutes in sugar-free products.
   - They have a minimal impact on blood sugar levels and provide fewer calories than regular sugar. However, excessive consumption can cause gastrointestinal issues, such as gas and diarrhea.
3. **Stevia**:
   - Stevia is a natural sweetener derived from the leaves of the Stevia rebaudiana plant. It is considered safe and does not raise blood sugar levels.
   - Stevia is available in various forms, including liquid drops and granulated versions, making it a versatile option for sweetening foods and beverages.
4. **Monk Fruit Extract**:

- Monk fruit extract is another natural sweetener derived from the monk fruit. It contains natural compounds called mogrosides, which are intensely sweet but do not affect blood sugar levels.
- Monk fruit extract is available in liquid, powder, and granulated forms.

5. **Agave Nectar**:
   - Agave nectar is a natural sweetener derived from the agave plant. It has a low glycemic index compared to regular sugar but is still a source of carbohydrates and calories.
   - Individuals with diabetes should use agave nectar sparingly and monitor its impact on blood sugar.

6. **Honey and Maple Syrup**:
   - While honey and maple syrup are natural sweeteners, they are high in carbohydrates and sugars. They can cause rapid increases in blood sugar and should be consumed in moderation by people with diabetes.

It's important to note that individual responses to sweeteners can vary. Some people may experience cravings or find that artificial sweeteners affect their taste preferences. Others may prefer to use small amounts of natural sweeteners in their diet. As with all aspects of diabetes management, it's essential to monitor your blood sugar levels and consult with a healthcare provider or registered dietitian to determine which sweeteners work best for you and align with your diabetes management plan. Additionally, it's a good practice to read food labels carefully to identify hidden sources of sweeteners and understand their potential impact on your blood sugar.

ALCOHOL AND DIABETES

Alcohol consumption can have both short-term and long-term effects on individuals with diabetes. It's important to be aware of how alcohol can impact blood sugar levels and overall health. Here are some key considerations regarding alcohol and diabetes:

1. **Effect on Blood Sugar**:

- Alcohol can lower blood sugar levels shortly after consumption, but it can also lead to delayed hypoglycemia (low blood sugar) several hours later.
- The liver processes alcohol before it processes glucose, which can result in hypoglycemia if you've taken diabetes medications that lower blood sugar, like insulin or certain oral medications.

2. **Carbohydrate Content**:
   - Some alcoholic beverages contain carbohydrates and can raise blood sugar levels. For example, beer, wine, and sweet cocktails contain sugars that can affect your glucose levels.

3. **Moderation is Key**:
   - If you choose to consume alcohol, do so in moderation. The American Diabetes Association recommends that women limit alcohol to one drink per day, and men to two drinks per day.
   - A standard drink is typically defined as 12 ounces of beer, 5 ounces of wine, or 1.5 ounces of distilled spirits.

4. **Impact of Mixed Drinks**:
   - Be cautious with mixed drinks, as they often contain added sugars and may significantly affect blood sugar levels.

5. **Check Blood Sugar**:
   - Monitor your blood sugar levels before, during, and after consuming alcohol to understand how it affects your body.

6. **Hypoglycemia Risk**:
   - Avoid drinking on an empty stomach. Consuming alcohol with a meal or a snack can help reduce the risk of hypoglycemia.

7. **Alcohol and Medications**:
   - Alcohol can interact with some diabetes medications and affect their effectiveness. Talk to your healthcare provider about how alcohol may interact with your specific medications.

8. **Stay Hydrated**:
   - Alcohol can lead to dehydration. Drink plenty of water alongside alcoholic beverages to stay well-hydrated.

9. **Alcohol and Complications**:

- Excessive alcohol consumption can lead to a higher risk of diabetes-related complications, particularly when it comes to the heart and liver. Individuals with diabetes are already at an increased risk of these complications, so it's important to be cautious with alcohol.

10. **Alcohol and Hypoglycemia Awareness**:
- If you are prone to hypoglycemia, be particularly cautious with alcohol. Ensure that someone around you is aware of your diabetes and how to help in case of severe low blood sugar.

11. **Plan Ahead**:
- If you plan to drink alcohol, consider reducing your carbohydrate intake in your meal or snack before drinking. This can help compensate for the potential rise in blood sugar from alcoholic beverages.

12. **Alternative Drinks**:
- If you want to enjoy social occasions without alcohol, consider non-alcoholic or sugar-free beverages.

13. **Individual Tolerance**:
- Diabetes affects individuals differently, so pay attention to how alcohol affects your body and adjust your choices accordingly.

In summary, while alcohol can be consumed in moderation by individuals with diabetes, it's essential to be aware of its effects on blood sugar, the importance of moderation, and the potential interactions with diabetes medications. Always consult with your healthcare provider for personalized guidance on alcohol consumption and diabetes management.

UNDERSTANDING THE IMPACT OF ALCOHOL ON DIABETES

Alcohol can have various effects on individuals with diabetes, including both short-term and long-term impacts. Here's a more detailed understanding of how alcohol affects diabetes management:

The Complete Diabetes Diet After 50

SHORT-TERM EFFECTS:

1. **Hypoglycemia Risk**: Alcohol can lower blood sugar levels shortly after consumption, potentially leading to hypoglycemia, especially if you've taken diabetes medications like insulin or sulfonylureas. The liver processes alcohol before glucose, making it more likely for low blood sugar to occur.
2. **Blood Sugar Fluctuations**: Alcohol can initially raise blood sugar due to its carbohydrate content in some drinks, but it may cause a drop in blood sugar later. The effect can vary depending on the type and amount of alcohol consumed.
3. **Reduced Inhibition**: Alcohol can impair judgment and reduce inhibitions, which might lead to less careful monitoring of dietary choices and blood sugar levels.

LONG-TERM EFFECTS:

1. **Weight Gain**: Alcohol is calorie-dense, and excessive consumption can lead to weight gain. For people with diabetes, maintaining a healthy weight is essential for blood sugar control.
2. **Liver Function**: Chronic alcohol consumption can negatively impact liver function, potentially worsening the effect of diabetes medications and impairing glucose regulation.
3. **Heart Health**: While moderate alcohol consumption may have some heart-protective effects, excessive drinking can increase the risk of heart disease, which is a significant concern for individuals with diabetes.
4. **Neuropathy and Complications**: Alcohol abuse can contribute to nerve damage (neuropathy) in individuals with diabetes. Alcohol can also exacerbate complications such as kidney disease and eye problems.
5. **Hypertension**: Alcohol can raise blood pressure, and high blood pressure is a risk factor for heart disease and stroke, conditions individuals with diabetes are already at an increased risk of.
6. **Medication Interactions**: Alcohol can interact with certain diabetes medications, potentially affecting their effectiveness. It's essential to consult with a healthcare provider about the potential interactions.

PERSONAL VARIATION:

The impact of alcohol on diabetes varies from person to person. Factors such as the type of diabetes, overall health, medication regimen, and individual tolerance to alcohol can influence how it affects blood sugar levels and overall health.

MODERATION AND MONITORING:

For individuals with diabetes, moderation is key when it comes to alcohol consumption. It's important to:

- Limit alcohol to moderate levels as recommended by healthcare providers.
- Monitor blood sugar levels closely before, during, and after drinking.
- Avoid drinking on an empty stomach and choose healthier food options if alcohol is consumed.
- Be aware of how alcohol affects your body and adjust your diabetes management plan accordingly.

Ultimately, the decision to consume alcohol and how to do so should be made in consultation with a healthcare provider who can provide personalized guidance based on your specific health needs and diabetes management goals.

MODERATION AND SAFE DRINKING FOR INDIVIDUALS WITH DIABETES

Drinking alcohol in moderation can be safe for many individuals with diabetes, but it's essential to follow some guidelines to ensure your safety and maintain good blood sugar control. Here are some tips for practicing moderation and safe drinking:

1. **Consult Your Healthcare Provider**:
   - Before making any changes to your alcohol consumption, discuss your plans with your healthcare provider. They can

help you understand how alcohol may interact with your diabetes medications and offer personalized advice.

2. **Know Your Limits**:
   - Understand what constitutes moderate drinking. For most adults, moderate drinking is defined as up to one drink per day for women and up to two drinks per day for men. A standard drink is typically defined as 12 ounces of beer, 5 ounces of wine, or 1.5 ounces of distilled spirits.

3. **Choose Low-Carb Options**:
   - When selecting alcoholic beverages, choose options that are lower in carbohydrates and sugars. For example, dry wines, light beers, and spirits with sugar-free mixers are better choices.

4. **Avoid High-Sugar Cocktails**:
   - Be cautious with cocktails that contain high-sugar mixers or syrups. These can cause rapid blood sugar spikes.

5. **Stay Hydrated**:
   - Alternate between alcoholic drinks and water to stay hydrated and help mitigate the dehydrating effects of alcohol.

6. **Don't Drink on an Empty Stomach**:
   - Consume alcohol with a meal or a snack to help stabilize your blood sugar levels. Avoid drinking on an empty stomach.

7. **Test Your Blood Sugar**:
   - Monitor your blood sugar levels before, during, and after drinking to track how alcohol affects your body. This helps you make informed decisions about your diabetes management.

8. **Limit Drinking Frequency**:
   - Even if you stay within the daily limits, limit the frequency of drinking to maintain good overall health.

9. **Understand Medication Interactions**:
   - Some diabetes medications can interact with alcohol, affecting blood sugar levels. Discuss these interactions with your healthcare provider.

10. **Prepare for Hypoglycemia**:

- Carry a source of fast-acting carbohydrates (like glucose tablets) in case you experience hypoglycemia. Alcohol can mask the symptoms of low blood sugar.

11. **Know When to Say No**:
- If you're unsure about the impact of alcohol on your blood sugar, it's better to abstain or choose non-alcoholic alternatives.

12. **Educate Your Social Circle**:
- Let your friends and family know about your diabetes and the importance of moderation in alcohol consumption. They can help support your choices.

13. **Avoid Drunk Driving**:
- Never drink and drive. Plan for a designated driver or alternative transportation if you'll be drinking.

14. **Monitor Your Health**:
- Regularly assess your overall health, including liver function, kidney function, and heart health. Diabetes can make you more vulnerable to the negative effects of excessive alcohol consumption.

Remember that the key to safe drinking for individuals with diabetes is moderation and awareness. Make informed decisions about when and how to consume alcohol and be prepared to adjust your diabetes management plan accordingly. Always consult with your healthcare provider for personalized advice and guidance on alcohol consumption in the context of your diabetes.

CHAPTER SEVEN
EATING OUT AND TRAVELING WITH DIABETES

Managing your diabetes while eating out or traveling can be challenging, but with some planning and strategies, you can enjoy these activities while maintaining good blood sugar control. Here are some tips for eating out and traveling with diabetes:

EATING OUT:

1. **Research the Menu in Advance**:
   - Many restaurants post their menus online. Review the menu before you go to choose options that align with your dietary needs and diabetes management plan.
2. **Choose Wisely**:
   - Look for dishes that are grilled, baked, broiled, or steamed, as these cooking methods generally involve less added fat. Opt for lean proteins, such as grilled chicken or fish.
3. **Control Portion Sizes**:
   - Restaurant portions are often larger than what you need. Consider sharing a dish or asking for a to-go container to save half for later.
4. **Ask for Modifications**:
   - Don't hesitate to request changes to your meal, such as substituting a side salad for fries or asking for sauces and dressings on the side.
5. **Avoid Sugary Drinks**:
   - Choose water, unsweetened tea, or diet beverages to avoid added sugars. Be mindful of alcohol consumption and choose lower-carb alcoholic drinks.
6. **Watch Carbohydrates**:
   - Be mindful of carbohydrate-heavy dishes like pasta, rice, and bread. Consider ordering extra vegetables or salad instead of these items.
7. **Monitor Blood Sugar**:

- Test your blood sugar levels before and after the meal to understand how the restaurant food affects your body.

8. **Be Prepared**:
   - Carry glucose tablets or snacks in case your blood sugar drops unexpectedly while dining out.

9. **Stay Mindful of Desserts**:
   - If you want to enjoy dessert, share it with a friend or family member to limit the portion size.

   TRAVELING:

1. **Pack Snacks**:
   - Bring diabetes-friendly snacks like nuts, seeds, and whole-grain crackers to have on hand when you're on the go.

2. **Carry Medications and Supplies**:
   - Ensure you have an adequate supply of medications, testing strips, and any necessary equipment. Pack extra in case of unexpected delays.

3. **Stay Hydrated**:
   - Travel can lead to dehydration. Drink plenty of water throughout your journey to stay hydrated.

4. **Adjust Meal Times**:
   - If you cross multiple time zones, work with your healthcare provider to adjust your meal and medication schedule as needed.

5. **Research Local Cuisine**:
   - Learn about the local foods and dishes you'll encounter in your travel destination. Understanding the ingredients and carbohydrate content can help you make informed choices.

6. **Eat Regular Meals**:
   - Try to stick to your regular meal schedule as much as possible to help maintain stable blood sugar levels.

7. **Be Prepared for Emergencies**:
   - Carry a card or wear a medical alert bracelet that indicates you have diabetes. This can be especially important when traveling in case of a medical emergency.

8. **Understand Local Healthcare**:
   - Research the availability of medical facilities and supplies at your destination in case you need them.

9. **Consult Your Healthcare Provider**:
    - Before traveling, discuss your plans with your healthcare provider. They can provide specific recommendations and guidance based on your individual health needs.

Eating out and traveling can still be enjoyable and manageable with diabetes. Planning ahead, making informed choices, and staying vigilant about your blood sugar levels are key components of successful diabetes management during these activities.

PHYSICAL ACTIVITY AND DIABETES

Physical activity is a crucial component of diabetes management, as it can help improve insulin sensitivity, lower blood sugar levels, and reduce the risk of diabetes-related complications. Here's how physical activity can benefit individuals with diabetes:

1. **Improved Insulin Sensitivity**:
    - Regular physical activity makes your cells more sensitive to insulin, allowing them to use glucose more efficiently. This can help lower blood sugar levels.
2. **Blood Sugar Control**:
    - Exercise helps lower blood sugar levels by increasing the uptake of glucose into muscle cells. It can also continue to have an impact on blood sugar levels for hours after you've finished exercising.
3. **Weight Management**:
    - Maintaining a healthy weight is important for diabetes management. Physical activity can help with weight loss or weight maintenance, which, in turn, can improve blood sugar control.
4. **Reduced Cardiovascular Risk**:
    - Diabetes is associated with an increased risk of heart disease. Regular exercise can help lower the risk of heart problems by improving cardiovascular health.
5. **Blood Pressure Control**:
    - Exercise can help lower high blood pressure, a common issue for people with diabetes.

6. **Cholesterol Management**:
   - Physical activity can raise "good" HDL cholesterol levels and lower "bad" LDL cholesterol levels, reducing the risk of heart disease.
7. **Stress Reduction**:
   - Exercise is a natural stress reliever, and managing stress can help control blood sugar levels.
8. **Better Sleep**:
   - Adequate sleep is essential for diabetes management. Regular physical activity can improve sleep quality.
9. **Improved Mood**:
   - Exercise releases endorphins, which can help improve your mood and reduce symptoms of depression or anxiety that can be associated with diabetes.
10. **Enhanced Muscle Strength and Flexibility**:
    - Strength training and flexibility exercises can help you build muscle, improve balance, and prevent falls, which can be important for older adults with diabetes.
11. **Overall Health Benefits**:
    - Exercise has numerous overall health benefits, including reducing the risk of chronic conditions like obesity, metabolic syndrome, and type 2 diabetes.

TO INCORPORATE PHYSICAL ACTIVITY INTO YOUR DIABETES MANAGEMENT PLAN:

1. **Consult Your Healthcare Provider**:
   - Before starting a new exercise regimen, talk to your healthcare provider to ensure that it's safe for your individual health needs and any potential complications related to your diabetes.
2. **Choose Activities You Enjoy**:
   - You're more likely to stick with an exercise routine if you enjoy the activities. Options can include walking, swimming, cycling, dancing, and more.
3. **Set Realistic Goals**:
   - Start with manageable goals and gradually increase the intensity and duration of your workouts. This approach helps prevent overexertion.

4. **Monitor Blood Sugar**:
   - Check your blood sugar levels before and after exercise to understand how different activities affect your body. Adjust your diabetes management plan as needed.
5. **Be Consistent**:
   - Aim for at least 150 minutes of moderate-intensity aerobic activity per week, along with muscle-strengthening activities on two or more days per week.
6. **Stay Hydrated**:
   - Drink plenty of water before, during, and after exercise.
7. **Include Warm-Up and Cool-Down**:
   - Always start with a warm-up and end with a cool-down to prevent injury.
8. **Consider Working with a Trainer or Physical Therapist**:
   - If you're unsure about how to start or have specific concerns, consider working with a professional who can help design an exercise plan tailored to your needs.
9. **Listen to Your Body**:
   - Pay attention to how your body responds to exercise. If you experience symptoms like dizziness, extreme fatigue, or severe fluctuations in blood sugar, stop the activity and seek medical advice.
10. **Stay Consistent**:
    - Make physical activity a regular part of your routine for the best long-term benefits.

Exercise is a powerful tool in diabetes management, but it's important to tailor your exercise routine to your individual needs and stay in close contact with your healthcare provider for guidance and adjustments.

CHAPTER EIGHT
MEDICATIONS AND INSULIN FOR DIABETES MANAGEMENT

Medications and insulin are essential components of diabetes management, especially for people with type 2 diabetes and some individuals with type 1 diabetes. They help control blood sugar levels and reduce the risk of diabetes-related complications. Here's an overview of common medications and insulin used in diabetes management:

FOR TYPE 1 DIABETES:

1. **Insulin**:
   - People with type 1 diabetes must take insulin because their bodies do not produce this hormone. There are several types of insulin, including:
     - **Rapid-Acting Insulin**: Begins working within 15 minutes and peaks in 1-2 hours.
     - **Short-Acting Insulin**: Starts working within 30 minutes and peaks in 2-3 hours.
     - **Intermediate-Acting Insulin**: Takes longer to start working (1-2 hours) and has a peak time of 4-12 hours.
     - **Long-Acting Insulin**: Provides a slow, steady release over 24 hours without a pronounced peak.

FOR TYPE 2 DIABETES:

1. **Oral Medications**:
   - There are several classes of oral medications that can be used alone or in combination to treat type 2 diabetes. Some common classes include:
     - **Metformin**: Improves insulin sensitivity and decreases the liver's glucose production.
     - **Sulfonylureas**: Stimulate the pancreas to release more insulin.

- **DPP-4 Inhibitors**: Increase insulin secretion and decrease glucagon production.
- **SGLT-2 Inhibitors**: Lower blood sugar levels by causing the kidneys to excrete excess glucose.
- **GLP-1 Receptor Agonists**: Increase insulin secretion, decrease glucagon production, and slow digestion to lower blood sugar.

2. **Injectable Medications**:
   - Some injectable medications are used in type 2 diabetes treatment, either alone or in combination with oral medications. These include GLP-1 receptor agonists and insulin.

3. **Insulin**:
   - In advanced cases or when other medications are no longer effective, people with type 2 diabetes may need to use insulin to manage their blood sugar levels. Insulin can be prescribed in various forms, similar to those used for type 1 diabetes.

OTHER DIABETES MEDICATIONS:

1. **Amylin Analogues**:
   - Amylin analogues mimic the effects of the hormone amylin, which helps control post-meal blood sugar spikes. These medications are often used in combination with insulin.

2. **Pramlintide**:
   - Pramlintide is an injectable medication that can be used in addition to insulin. It helps slow digestion, reducing post-meal blood sugar spikes.

3. **Medications for Blood Pressure and Cholesterol**:
   - Some individuals with diabetes may need medications to manage high blood pressure and cholesterol levels, which are risk factors for heart disease, a common complication of diabetes.

It's important to note that the choice of medication or insulin and the treatment plan is highly individualized. Your healthcare provider will consider your specific needs, lifestyle, and medical history when determining the best approach for you. Regular monitoring of blood sugar levels is also essential to ensure that your treatment plan is effective and to make necessary adjustments. Diabetes management is a collaborative effort between you and your healthcare team, so be sure to communicate your needs, concerns, and goals to your healthcare provider.

DIABETES MEDICATIONS AFTER 50

As individuals age, their healthcare needs and diabetes management may change. Here are some considerations for diabetes medications for people aged 50 and older:

1. **Individualized Treatment Plans**:
   - Diabetes management is not one-size-fits-all. As you age, your healthcare provider will continue to develop a personalized treatment plan that considers your overall health, medication tolerance, and lifestyle.
2. **Oral Medications**:
   - For people with type 2 diabetes, oral medications are commonly used. Medications such as metformin, sulfonylureas, DPP-4 inhibitors, and SGLT-2 inhibitors are often prescribed. Your healthcare provider may adjust your medication regimen to optimize blood sugar control while considering any age-related health issues.
3. **Glucose Monitoring**:
   - Regular blood glucose monitoring is essential. This helps your healthcare provider determine if your current medication regimen is effective and whether adjustments are necessary.
4. **Medication Adjustments**:
   - As you age, your body may become more sensitive to medications or may require different dosages. Your healthcare provider will monitor your response to medication and make adjustments as needed.
5. **Incretin-Based Therapies**:
   - GLP-1 receptor agonists, which enhance insulin secretion and reduce blood sugar levels, are often used in diabetes

management for older adults. They may also promote weight loss, which can be beneficial for older individuals.

6. **Safety and Side Effects**:
   - Older adults may be at greater risk for side effects or drug interactions due to the use of multiple medications. Work closely with your healthcare provider to manage potential risks.

7. **Blood Pressure and Cholesterol Medications**:
   - People with diabetes often require medications to manage blood pressure and cholesterol levels. As you age, these medications may become even more critical for heart health.

8. **Avoiding Hypoglycemia**:
   - Older adults are more prone to hypoglycemia (low blood sugar). Be cautious with medications that can increase this risk, especially if you're taking multiple medications.

9. **Kidney Function**:
   - Kidney function tends to decline with age, and some diabetes medications are processed by the kidneys. Your healthcare provider may adjust your medication regimen to accommodate any changes in kidney function.

10. **Comorbid Conditions**:
    - As you age, you may develop other health conditions in addition to diabetes. Your healthcare provider will consider how these conditions may impact your diabetes management and medication choices.

11. **Mental Health and Cognitive Function**:
    - Diabetes management can be complex, and older adults may face challenges related to cognitive function or mental health. It's important to address these issues with your healthcare provider and seek support if needed.

12. **Lifestyle Factors**:
    - Lifestyle modifications, such as diet and physical activity, remain crucial for diabetes management at any age. Discuss any changes in your lifestyle with your healthcare provider to ensure they align with your treatment plan.

13. **Vaccinations and Preventive Care**:

- Older adults with diabetes should stay up to date with vaccinations, including those for influenza and pneumonia, to reduce the risk of infections that can impact blood sugar control.

14. **Regular Health Checkups**:
    - Stay committed to regular checkups with your healthcare provider, who will continue to assess your overall health and provide guidance on managing your diabetes.

Diabetes management can be successful at any age, but it requires ongoing communication with your healthcare provider, medication adjustments, and a commitment to a healthy lifestyle. As you age, it's important to adapt your diabetes management plan to meet your changing needs and maintain good blood sugar control.

INSULIN MANAGEMENT FOR DIABETES

Insulin is a crucial hormone for individuals with diabetes, particularly those with type 1 diabetes and some with type 2 diabetes. Proper insulin management is essential for maintaining stable blood sugar levels and preventing diabetes-related complications. Here are some key considerations for insulin management:

1. Consult with a Healthcare Provider:

- Work closely with your healthcare provider, such as an endocrinologist or diabetes specialist, to create an individualized insulin management plan that considers your specific needs, lifestyle, and goals.

2. Types of Insulin:

- There are various types of insulin with different characteristics:
    - **Rapid-Acting Insulin**: Begins working within 15 minutes and is taken just before or after meals.

- **Short-Acting Insulin**: Starts working within 30 minutes and is taken about 30 minutes before meals.
- **Intermediate-Acting Insulin**: Has a slower onset and a longer duration, often taken once or twice a day.
- **Long-Acting Insulin**: Provides a steady release of insulin over 24 hours and is taken once a day.

3. Insulin Delivery Methods:

- Insulin can be delivered through various methods, including insulin injections using syringes or insulin pens, and insulin pumps. The choice of delivery method depends on your preferences and your healthcare provider's recommendations.

4. Timing and Dosage:

- Follow your healthcare provider's guidance regarding when to take insulin and the correct dosage for each type. Consistency is key to maintaining stable blood sugar levels.

5. Monitoring Blood Sugar:

- Regularly monitor your blood sugar levels using a glucose meter. This helps you adjust your insulin doses as needed and provides valuable information for your healthcare provider.

6. Carbohydrate Counting:

- If you're taking mealtime insulin, you may be taught how to count carbohydrates to match your insulin doses with your meal choices. This can help you better manage your blood sugar.

7. Hypoglycemia Awareness:

- Be aware of the signs and symptoms of hypoglycemia (low blood sugar) and how to treat it with glucose tablets or snacks. Carry supplies for treating low blood sugar with you at all times.

8. Hyperglycemia Management:

- Understand how to manage hyperglycemia (high blood sugar) as well. Your healthcare provider will provide guidance on when and how to adjust your insulin doses when blood sugar levels are elevated.

9. Injection Site Rotation:

- If you're using injections, rotate the injection sites to prevent lipodystrophy (fat tissue changes) and ensure consistent insulin absorption.

10. Lifestyle Factors: - Adjust your insulin doses based on your daily activities, such as exercise, meals, and changes in routine. Be prepared to make adjustments with your healthcare provider's guidance.

11. Storage and Handling: - Insulin should be stored properly according to the manufacturer's instructions. Check the expiration dates and ensure that the insulin is not exposed to extreme temperatures.

12. Travel Considerations: - When traveling, be prepared with enough insulin and supplies for the duration of your trip. Know how to manage time zone changes and meal schedules.

13. Regular Checkups: - Continue with regular checkups and consultations with your healthcare provider to assess your insulin management plan and make any necessary adjustments.

14. Emergency Preparedness: - Have an emergency plan in case of insulin supply disruptions or natural disasters. Keep extra insulin and supplies on hand when possible.

Effective insulin management is essential for controlling blood sugar levels and preventing diabetes-related complications. Be proactive in managing your diabetes, stay in close communication with your healthcare provider, and stay informed about the latest advancements in diabetes management and insulin therapy.

CHAPTER NINE
BLOOD SUGAR MONITORING FOR DIABETES

Regular blood sugar monitoring is a fundamental aspect of managing diabetes. It provides valuable information about your blood glucose levels, enabling you to make informed decisions about your diet, physical activity, and medication. Here's a guide to blood sugar monitoring for individuals with diabetes:

1. Frequency of Monitoring:

- The frequency of blood sugar monitoring can vary based on your type of diabetes, treatment plan, and individual circumstances. Some individuals may need to monitor multiple times a day, while others may only need to check a few times a week. Work with your healthcare provider to determine the appropriate frequency for you.

2. Timing of Monitoring:

The timing of blood sugar checks can include:
- Fasting: In the morning before eating (often to assess overnight blood sugar levels).
- Before meals: To determine pre-meal glucose levels.
- After meals: To understand how different foods affect your blood sugar.
- Bedtime: To ensure blood sugar levels are stable overnight.
- Before and after exercise: To gauge the impact of physical activity.

3. Glucose Monitoring Devices:

There are various devices for blood sugar monitoring, including:
- **Glucose Meters**: Handheld devices that require a drop of blood from a fingerstick. They provide immediate results.

- **Continuous Glucose Monitors (CGMs)**: These wearable devices continuously measure glucose levels and provide real-time data, including trends and patterns.
- **Flash Glucose Monitoring**: A variation of CGMs that doesn't require constant sensor-to-reader contact.
- **Urine Test Strips**: Less common today, they provide a general idea of glucose levels but are less precise than blood-based monitoring.

4. Blood Sample Collection:

- For glucose meters and CGMs, you typically collect a small blood sample by pricking your finger using a lancet. Follow the manufacturer's instructions for proper blood sample collection.

5. Record Keeping:

- Maintain a blood sugar log to track your readings, medications, meals, physical activity, and other relevant information. This log can help you and your healthcare provider identify patterns and adjust your diabetes management plan as needed.

6. Target Blood Sugar Levels:

- Work with your healthcare provider to establish target blood sugar ranges for fasting, pre-meal, post-meal, and bedtime readings. These targets are individualized and may change over time.

7. Hypoglycemia (Low Blood Sugar):

- Be aware of the symptoms of hypoglycemia, such as shakiness, sweating, and confusion. Test your blood sugar when you experience these symptoms and treat accordingly.

8. Hyperglycemia (High Blood Sugar):

- Understand the signs of hyperglycemia, like extreme thirst and frequent urination. Test your blood sugar if you experience these symptoms and take action according to your healthcare provider's guidance.

9. Trends and Patterns:

- Use your blood sugar data to identify trends and patterns. For instance, you might notice that your blood sugar is consistently high after certain meals. This information can inform adjustments to your diet or medication.

10. Regular Check-Ins: - Share your blood sugar log with your healthcare provider during regular check-ups. They can assess your progress and help you make necessary adjustments to your diabetes management plan.

11. Seek Professional Guidance: - Always consult with your healthcare provider for guidance on blood sugar monitoring and diabetes management. They can provide personalized advice based on your specific health needs and goals.

Blood sugar monitoring is a powerful tool that empowers individuals with diabetes to take control of their health. It allows for timely interventions, promotes better blood sugar control, and reduces the risk of complications. Regular communication with your healthcare provider is essential to ensure that your monitoring plan aligns with your overall diabetes management strategy.

THE IMPORTANCE OF REGULAR BLOOD SUGAR TESTING IN DIABETES MANAGEMENT

Regular blood sugar testing is a cornerstone of effective diabetes management. It provides critical information about your blood glucose levels, allowing you to make informed decisions and adjustments to your treatment plan. Here's why regular testing is so important for individuals with diabetes:

1. Individualized Care: Diabetes is a highly individualized condition. What works for one person may not work for another. Regular blood sugar testing enables your healthcare provider to tailor your treatment plan to your specific needs, lifestyle, and goals.

2. Blood Sugar Awareness: Testing helps you become more aware of how your body responds to different factors, such as meals, exercise, stress, and medications. This awareness allows you to take proactive steps to manage your condition effectively.

3. Monitoring for Hypoglycemia: Regular testing helps you detect and address hypoglycemia (low blood sugar) promptly. Hypoglycemia can be dangerous and cause symptoms like shakiness, confusion, and, in severe cases, unconsciousness. Testing allows you to take quick action to raise your blood sugar levels when needed.

4. Preventing Hyperglycemia: Hyperglycemia (high blood sugar) is a significant concern in diabetes, as it can lead to long-term complications. Regular testing helps identify high blood sugar levels so that you can take appropriate steps to lower them.

5. Medication Adjustment: For individuals taking diabetes medications, including insulin, regular testing is essential for determining the appropriate dosages and timing. If you notice consistent patterns of high or low blood sugar, your healthcare provider can make medication adjustments accordingly.

6. Lifestyle Modifications: Blood sugar testing is a valuable tool for evaluating the impact of dietary choices and physical activity on your glucose levels. This information can guide dietary changes, meal planning, and exercise routines.

7. Goal Setting: Your healthcare provider will set target blood sugar ranges for different times of the day (e.g., fasting, pre-meal, post-meal) based on your individual needs. Regular testing helps you gauge your progress toward these goals.

8. Prevention of Complications: Uncontrolled diabetes can lead to a range of complications, including heart disease, kidney problems, eye issues, and nerve damage. Regular blood sugar monitoring is a key element in reducing the risk of these complications.

9. Data Analysis: Over time, blood sugar data can reveal trends and patterns that inform your diabetes management. You might discover that your blood sugar consistently rises after consuming certain foods or under specific circumstances. This knowledge empowers you to make informed decisions about your diet and lifestyle.

10. Improved Quality of Life: Effective diabetes management helps you feel better, maintain your energy levels, and enjoy a higher quality of life. Regular testing plays a crucial role in achieving these outcomes.

11. Accountability: Regular testing helps you stay accountable to your diabetes management plan. It provides concrete evidence of your progress and areas that may need attention, encouraging you to stay on track.

12. Education and Empowerment: Blood sugar testing is an educational tool. It helps you understand the direct impact of your choices on your health, empowering you to take control of your diabetes.

13. Communication with Healthcare Providers: Your healthcare provider relies on your blood sugar data to assess your diabetes management and make recommendations for adjustments. Regular check-ins with your healthcare team are essential for long-term success.

In summary, regular blood sugar testing is a fundamental aspect of diabetes management. It provides insights, awareness, and the information needed to make informed decisions about your health.

By monitoring your blood sugar levels consistently, you can take proactive steps to achieve good blood sugar control, reduce the risk of complications, and lead a healthier life with diabetes.

INTERPRETING BLOOD SUGAR RESULTS IN DIABETES

Interpreting blood sugar results is a crucial aspect of diabetes management. Understanding the meaning of your blood sugar readings allows you to make informed decisions about your diet, medication, and overall health. Here's a guide to help you interpret blood sugar results effectively:

1. Target Blood Sugar Ranges:

- Start by establishing target blood sugar ranges with your healthcare provider. These targets will vary depending on your type of diabetes, age, and overall health. Common target ranges include:
    - Fasting (before meals): Typically 80-130 mg/dL (4.4-7.2 mmol/L).
    - Post-meal (1-2 hours after eating): Generally below 180 mg/dL (10 mmol/L).

2. Fasting Blood Sugar:

- Fasting blood sugar is typically measured in the morning before eating or drinking anything. A reading within your target range is a positive sign that your overnight blood sugar control is on track.
- **Interpretation**:
    - Within Target Range: Good blood sugar control.
    - Above Target Range: May indicate the need for dietary or medication adjustments.
    - Below Target Range: May suggest overmedication or other issues; consult your healthcare provider.

3. Post-Meal Blood Sugar:

- Post-meal blood sugar levels are measured 1-2 hours after eating. These readings provide insight into how your body processes the glucose from meals.
- **Interpretation**:
    - Within Target Range: Suggests effective meal planning and blood sugar control.
    - Above Target Range: May indicate that your meals are causing blood sugar spikes. Consider modifying your diet or medication.
    - Below Target Range: Uncommon but may be due to rapid-acting medication. Consult your healthcare provider.

4. Continuous Glucose Monitoring (CGM) Trends:

- CGMs provide a continuous stream of glucose data. Pay attention to trends over hours or days to identify patterns. Look for fluctuations, spikes, and dips in your glucose levels.
- **Interpretation**:
    - Consistent within Target Range: Indicates stable blood sugar control.
    - Frequent Spikes: May require dietary or medication adjustments.
    - Frequent Dips: Suggests potential issues with insulin or medication dosages. Consult your healthcare provider.

5. Hypoglycemia (Low Blood Sugar):

- Low blood sugar, or hypoglycemia, can occur when your levels drop below your target range, typically below 70 mg/dL (3.9 mmol/L). Symptoms may include shakiness, confusion, and sweating.
- **Interpretation**:
    - Low Blood Sugar: Address immediately with a fast-acting carbohydrate source, such as glucose tablets, to raise your blood sugar back into the target range.
    - Frequent Hypoglycemia: Consult your healthcare provider to identify the cause and make necessary adjustments.

6. Hyperglycemia (High Blood Sugar):

- High blood sugar, or hyperglycemia, occurs when your levels rise above your target range. Symptoms may include excessive thirst, frequent urination, and fatigue.
- **Interpretation**:
    - High Blood Sugar: Take action according to your healthcare provider's guidance, such as adjusting your medication, increasing physical activity, or modifying your diet.
    - Frequent Hyperglycemia: Consult your healthcare provider for adjustments to your diabetes management plan.

7. Consistency and Trends:

- Pay attention to the overall consistency of your blood sugar readings and look for trends over time. If you notice recurring patterns of high or low blood sugar, discuss these with your healthcare provider.

8. Consult Your Healthcare Provider:

- Regularly share your blood sugar data with your healthcare provider during check-ups. They can analyze your results and provide guidance on managing your diabetes effectively.

9. Adjustments and Personalization:

- Remember that diabetes management is highly individualized. Your healthcare provider will work with you to adjust your treatment plan as needed to maintain stable blood sugar control.

10. Emotional Well-Being: - Lastly, consider the emotional impact of your blood sugar readings. Fluctuations can be frustrating or concerning, but remember that these readings are tools to help you manage your condition, not measures of your self-worth.

Interpreting blood sugar results requires careful consideration of your individual targets and an understanding of the factors that can influence your readings. Regular communication with your healthcare provider is key to ensuring that your diabetes management plan remains effective and aligned with your unique needs and goals.

CHAPTER TEN
MANAGING DIABETES COMPLICATIONS

Living with diabetes requires proactive management to prevent and manage complications. Over time, uncontrolled blood sugar levels can lead to various health issues. Here are some key steps to effectively manage diabetes complications:

1. Regular Medical Check-Ups:

- Attend regular check-ups with your healthcare provider. These visits allow for the early detection and management of diabetes-related complications.

2. Blood Pressure Control:

- High blood pressure (hypertension) is a common complication of diabetes and a risk factor for heart disease and kidney problems. Work with your healthcare provider to keep your blood pressure in a healthy range.

3. Cholesterol Management:

- High levels of "bad" LDL cholesterol and low levels of "good" HDL cholesterol can increase the risk of heart disease. Managing cholesterol levels is vital. Discuss medication options and dietary changes with your healthcare provider.

4. Kidney Health:

- Diabetes is a leading cause of kidney disease. Regular kidney function tests, such as estimated glomerular filtration rate (eGFR) and urinary albumin-to-creatinine ratio, can help monitor kidney health.

5. Eye Exams:

- Diabetes can damage the blood vessels in the eyes, leading to diabetic retinopathy, a common cause of vision loss. Regular eye exams can detect issues early when they're most treatable.

6. Foot Care:

- Neuropathy (nerve damage) and poor circulation can lead to foot problems in people with diabetes. Inspect your feet daily for any cuts, sores, or blisters, and wear comfortable shoes. Regular podiatry check-ups are important.

7. Dental and Gum Health:

- Diabetes can increase the risk of gum disease. Good oral hygiene and regular dental check-ups can help prevent oral health problems.

8. Neuropathy Management:

- Diabetic neuropathy can cause pain, numbness, and tingling in the extremities. Medications and lifestyle changes can help manage symptoms. Regularly inspect your skin and feet for any issues.

9. Weight Management:

- Maintaining a healthy weight is crucial for overall diabetes management. If you're overweight, losing even a modest amount of weight can improve blood sugar control and reduce the risk of complications.

10. Blood Sugar Control: - The cornerstone of diabetes management is controlling blood sugar levels. Work with your healthcare provider to establish target ranges for fasting, pre-meal, and post-meal blood sugar readings. Regular monitoring and adjustments to your treatment plan are essential.

11. Lifestyle Modifications: - Adopt a healthy lifestyle that includes a balanced diet, regular physical activity, stress management, and adequate sleep. These factors can help manage blood sugar and reduce complications.

12. Medication Adherence: - Take your diabetes medications as prescribed. Skipping doses or not following your medication plan can lead to uncontrolled blood sugar levels and complications.

13. Support Networks: - Join support groups or seek the help of a mental health professional if you're struggling with the emotional aspects of managing diabetes. Emotional well-being is an important component of overall health.

14. Diabetes Education: - Consider enrolling in diabetes education programs. They can provide valuable information and strategies for managing your condition effectively.

15. Emergency Preparedness: - Always have a plan for managing your diabetes during emergencies, such as natural disasters. Ensure you have an adequate supply of medications and necessary supplies.

16. Collaborate with Your Healthcare Team: - Work closely with your healthcare provider and a team of specialists, as needed, to manage your diabetes and any related complications. Regular communication is essential.

Managing diabetes complications requires a proactive and comprehensive approach. By prioritizing regular check-ups, blood sugar control, and a healthy lifestyle, you can reduce the risk of complications and lead a fulfilling life with diabetes. Remember that early detection and intervention are key to effective management.

SUPPORT SYSTEMS FOR MANAGING DIABETES

Living with diabetes can be challenging, and having a strong support system is crucial for effective management and emotional well-being. Here are various sources of support that can help individuals with diabetes:

1. Healthcare Team:

- Your healthcare provider, such as an endocrinologist or primary care physician, plays a central role in your diabetes management. Regular check-ups and open communication are essential for optimizing your treatment plan.

2. Diabetes Educators:

- Certified diabetes educators can provide guidance on diabetes self-management, including medication, diet, exercise, and blood sugar monitoring.

3. Registered Dietitians/Nutritionists:

- Nutrition professionals can help you create a personalized meal plan that aligns with your dietary preferences and diabetes management goals.

4. Mental Health Professionals:

- Psychologists, counselors, or therapists can offer emotional support and coping strategies for dealing with the psychological aspects of diabetes.

5. Support Groups:

- Joining a diabetes support group can connect you with others who understand the daily challenges of living with diabetes. Sharing experiences and strategies can be comforting and educational.

6. Family and Friends:

- Loved ones can provide invaluable emotional support and encouragement. Share your diabetes management goals and needs with them to foster understanding and empathy.

7. Online Communities:

- Online forums, social media groups, and websites dedicated to diabetes offer a platform for sharing experiences and gaining insights from a diverse community of individuals managing diabetes.

8. Diabetes Apps and Technology:

- Utilize diabetes management apps and wearable technology to track blood sugar, medication, diet, and exercise. These tools can provide valuable data and reminders.

9. Diabetes Organizations:

- National and local diabetes association's often offer educational resources, events, and support services. These organizations can help you stay informed and connected.

10. Pharmacist: - Your pharmacist can offer guidance on diabetes medications, including proper administration and potential side effects.

11. Work or School Support: - Inform your employer or school about your diabetes, and work together to create a supportive environment. This may involve accommodations or adjustments to your schedule or workspace.

12. Religious or Spiritual Communities: - Faith-based communities can provide emotional and spiritual support, as well as opportunities for outreach and assistance.

13. Exercise and Fitness Professionals: - Certified trainers or physical therapists can help you design safe and effective exercise routines tailored to your diabetes management needs.

14. Online Resources: - Numerous websites and apps offer educational materials, diabetes management tools, and healthy living tips.

15. Financial Counselors: - Managing the costs of diabetes care can be a concern. Financial counselors or social workers can provide assistance in navigating insurance, prescription assistance programs, and other financial resources.

16. Diabetes Camps and Retreats: - Attending diabetes-focused camps or retreats can provide a sense of community and empowerment while learning more about managing diabetes.

17. Diabetes Advocacy Groups: - Joining or supporting diabetes advocacy organizations can help raise awareness and promote policies that benefit people with diabetes.

18. Spouse or Caregiver Support: - If you are caring for someone with diabetes, ensure you have the knowledge and resources to assist them effectively.

19. Cultural or Community Groups: - Engage with cultural or community organizations that may provide culturally sensitive resources and support.

A strong support system can make a significant difference in your ability to manage diabetes effectively. It's important to reach out to these sources of support and engage with the ones that best fit your needs and preferences. Remember that you are not alone in your journey with diabetes, and there are many individuals and organizations ready to assist you.

BUILDING A DIABETES CARE TEAM

Effective diabetes management often requires a multidisciplinary approach, involving various healthcare professionals with specialized knowledge and skills. Building a diabetes care team can help you receive comprehensive care and support. Here are the key members to consider including in your diabetes care team:

1. Primary Care Physician:

- Your primary care doctor is often the first point of contact for diabetes management. They can help with diagnosis, general care, and referrals to specialists when needed.

2. Endocrinologist:

- An endocrinologist is a medical doctor who specializes in hormones and endocrine disorders, including diabetes. They can provide in-depth knowledge and treatment for diabetes.

3. Certified Diabetes Educator (CDE):

- CDEs are healthcare professionals who specialize in teaching individuals with diabetes how to manage their condition. They can provide education on self-care, nutrition, medications, and more.

4. Registered Dietitian or Nutritionist:

- A registered dietitian or nutritionist can help you create a personalized meal plan to manage your blood sugar levels and maintain a balanced diet.

5. Ophthalmologist or Optometrist:

- Regular eye exams are essential for monitoring and preventing diabetes-related eye complications, such as diabetic retinopathy.

6. Dentist or Periodontist:

- Diabetes can increase the risk of gum disease, so regular dental check-ups are important for oral health.

7. Cardiologist:

- If you have cardiovascular risk factors or existing heart disease, a cardiologist can provide specialized care and monitoring.

8. Podiatrist:

- Foot care is crucial for people with diabetes to prevent complications. A podiatrist specializes in foot and ankle health.

9. Mental Health Professional:

- A psychologist, counselor, or therapist can help you address the emotional and psychological aspects of living with diabetes.

10. Pharmacist: - Your pharmacist can provide information on diabetes medications, help with medication management, and address questions or concerns.

11. Exercise Specialist: - A certified personal trainer or physical therapist can assist in designing and implementing an exercise plan tailored to your specific needs and fitness level.

12. Social Worker: - Social workers can help you navigate social and financial challenges related to diabetes, such as accessing support programs or dealing with insurance.

13. Diabetes Nurse Specialist: - A diabetes nurse specialist is a registered nurse with specialized training in diabetes care. They can provide education, guidance, and support.

14. Diabetes Care Team Coordinator: - This individual, often found in larger healthcare systems, can help coordinate and facilitate communication among various members of your care team.

15. Support Group Leader: - Support groups are often led by individuals with diabetes or healthcare professionals and can offer peer support, information, and resources.

16. Health Technology Expert: - As technology plays an increasingly important role in diabetes management, consider involving an expert who can help you with devices, apps, and monitoring tools.

Building your diabetes care team should be a collaborative effort. Your primary care physician or endocrinologist can help you identify the specific team members you need based on your unique health needs and goals. Effective communication and coordination among your care team members are essential to ensure that your diabetes management plan is well-coordinated and comprehensive.

EMOTIONAL WELLBEING AND DIABETES

Emotional wellbeing is a vital aspect of diabetes management, as living with diabetes can be challenging both physically and emotionally. It's important to address the psychological and emotional impact of diabetes to ensure overall well-being. Here are some key considerations for maintaining emotional health while managing diabetes:

1. Self-Awareness:

- Recognize and acknowledge your emotions, including frustration, anxiety, stress, and even grief. It's normal to have a range of feelings when living with a chronic condition.

2. Support System:

- Build a strong support system that includes friends, family, support groups, or a mental health professional. Sharing your feelings with others who understand can be comforting and empowering.

3. Diabetes Education:

- Educate yourself about diabetes and its management. Understanding your condition can reduce anxiety and fear.

4. Stress Management:

- Practice stress-reduction techniques, such as mindfulness, meditation, deep breathing, or progressive muscle relaxation. These methods can help you manage stress and anxiety.

5. Regular Physical Activity:

- Exercise is not only beneficial for physical health but also for mental well-being. It can reduce stress, improve mood, and boost self-esteem.

6. Healthy Diet:

- Proper nutrition can influence mood and energy levels. A balanced diet can help stabilize blood sugar and improve overall well-being.

7. Medication Adherence:

- Take your diabetes medications as prescribed. Uncontrolled blood sugar levels can lead to mood swings and emotional distress.

8. Set Realistic Goals:

- Establish achievable goals for diabetes management and life in general. Success in reaching these goals can boost your self-esteem.

9. Celebrate Achievements:

- Acknowledge and celebrate your successes, no matter how small. Reward yourself for meeting your goals and managing your diabetes effectively.

10. Seek Professional Help: - If you're struggling with emotional distress or mental health issues related to diabetes, don't hesitate to consult a psychologist, counselor, or therapist. They can provide tools to cope with stress and anxiety.

11. Communicate with Your Healthcare Team: - Open and honest communication with your healthcare provider is crucial. They can address your concerns and help you make necessary adjustments to your treatment plan.

12. Balance Information: - While staying informed is essential, avoid overwhelming yourself with constant research and information about diabetes. Balance knowledge with personal well-being.

13. Mindful Eating: - Pay attention to your eating habits and emotional eating triggers. Food should nourish your body, not be used as a coping mechanism.

14. Diabetes Management Tools: - Utilize technology and tools, such as blood glucose meters, insulin pumps, or continuous glucose monitors, to make diabetes management more manageable.

15. Routine and Consistency: - Establish daily routines for blood sugar monitoring, medication administration, and meal planning. Consistency can reduce stress.

16. Acceptance: - Accept that diabetes is a part of your life, but it doesn't define you. Embrace your condition and take control of your health.

17. Diabetes Support Groups: - Consider joining a local or online diabetes support group to connect with others who share similar experiences and challenges.

18. Advocate for Yourself: - Be an advocate for your health by speaking up and asking questions during medical appointments. Ensure that your concerns are addressed.

19. Positive Self-Talk: - Replace negative self-talk with positive affirmations and self-compassion. Treat yourself with kindness and understanding.

Emotional wellbeing is a fundamental aspect of managing diabetes effectively. By taking care of your mental health, you can better cope with the challenges that diabetes presents and lead a fulfilling life. Remember that it's okay to seek help and support when needed, and you don't have to face diabetes alone.

CHAPTER ELEVEN
DIABETES AND AGING

Diabetes is a chronic condition that can impact people of all ages, but its management and effects can change as individuals age. Here are some key considerations related to diabetes and aging:

1. Increased Risk: The risk of developing type 2 diabetes increases with age. This is partly due to factors like decreased physical activity, changes in metabolism, and potential genetic predisposition. It's essential for older adults to monitor their health and stay vigilant for signs of diabetes.

2. Complications:

- Diabetes can lead to a range of complications, including heart disease, kidney problems, nerve damage, vision issues, and more. Older adults are often at greater risk for these complications due to the cumulative impact of diabetes on the body over time.

3. Cognitive Health:

- There is evidence to suggest a connection between diabetes and cognitive decline, including an increased risk of dementia. Maintaining good blood sugar control is vital to reduce this risk.

4. Medication Management:

- Older adults often take multiple medications for various health conditions. It's important to manage these medications carefully, as some can interact with diabetes medications or affect blood sugar levels.

5. Blood Sugar Control:

- Achieving and maintaining good blood sugar control is essential for older adults with diabetes. Proper control can help prevent complications and improve overall health.

6. Hypoglycemia (Low Blood Sugar):

- Older adults are at an increased risk of hypoglycemia, which can have serious consequences. It's crucial to monitor blood sugar levels regularly and be aware of the signs of low blood sugar.

7. Heart Health:

- Cardiovascular health is a significant concern for older adults with diabetes. High blood pressure and cholesterol levels can compound the risk of heart disease. Maintaining a heart-healthy lifestyle and working closely with healthcare providers to manage risk factors are essential.

8. Physical Activity:

- Staying physically active remains important for older adults with diabetes. It can help with blood sugar control, weight management, and overall well-being.

9. Nutrition:

- A balanced diet is crucial for older adults with diabetes. Dietary choices play a significant role in blood sugar management and overall health.

10. Regular Check-Ups: - Older adults with diabetes should have regular check-ups with their healthcare provider to monitor their diabetes, manage medications, and address any potential complications.

11. Emotional Wellbeing: - The emotional impact of managing diabetes can be significant. Emotional health is essential for overall well-being, and older adults should seek support and resources to help cope with the challenges of diabetes.

12. Support System: - A strong support system is valuable for older adults with diabetes. Family, friends, support groups, and healthcare providers can provide guidance, encouragement, and assistance.

13. Lifestyle Adjustments: - As individuals age, they may need to make adjustments to their lifestyle and diabetes management plan to accommodate changing health needs and capabilities.

14. Diabetes Education: - Staying informed about diabetes and its management is essential. Diabetes education programs can provide valuable information and support for older adults.

15. Individualized Care: - Diabetes management is highly individualized. Older adults should work closely with their healthcare team to develop a care plan that meets their unique needs and goals.

16. Prevention: - Older adults can reduce their risk of developing diabetes by adopting a healthy lifestyle that includes regular physical activity, a balanced diet, and maintaining a healthy weight.

Managing diabetes in older age requires attention to various factors, including health, lifestyle, and emotional well-being. By staying informed, seeking support, and working closely with healthcare providers, older adults can effectively manage their diabetes and enjoy a good quality of life as they age.

COPING WITH THE CHALLENGES OF AGING WITH DIABETES

Aging with diabetes presents unique challenges that require proactive management and a positive outlook. Here are some strategies to help you cope effectively with these challenges:

1. Stay Informed:

- Continue to educate yourself about diabetes, its management, and the potential complications associated with aging. Knowledge is empowering and helps you make informed decisions.

2. Regular Check-Ups:

- Consistent healthcare check-ups are essential. Regularly monitor your blood sugar, blood pressure, cholesterol, and other vital health markers. These check-ups help in early detection and management of any issues.

3. Medication Management:

- If you take multiple medications for various conditions, consider using pill organizers or medication management apps to ensure you take the right doses at the right times.

4. Balanced Diet:

- Focus on a balanced and nutritious diet that suits your specific health needs. Consult a registered dietitian to create a meal plan that helps manage your diabetes while meeting your nutritional requirements.

5. Physical Activity:

- Engage in regular physical activity that is appropriate for your fitness level and health condition. Activities like walking, swimming, or low-impact exercises can improve blood sugar control and overall well-being.

6. Blood Sugar Monitoring:

- Monitor your blood sugar levels regularly, especially if you take insulin or other medications that can cause hypoglycemia. Keep glucose tablets or fast-acting carbohydrates on hand in case of low blood sugar.

7. Hypoglycemia Awareness:

- Be aware of the signs and symptoms of hypoglycemia (low blood sugar). Older adults are at higher risk, so early recognition is crucial for prompt treatment.

8. Heart Health:

- Pay attention to heart health by managing blood pressure and cholesterol levels. A heart-healthy lifestyle can reduce the risk of heart disease, a common complication of diabetes.

9. Cognitive Health:

- Engage in activities that support cognitive health, such as puzzles, reading, and social interaction. Managing blood sugar levels and staying physically active can also benefit cognitive function.

10. Medication Adherence: - Ensure that you take your diabetes medications as prescribed. Consult your healthcare provider if you experience any side effects or have difficulty managing your medications.

11. Emotional Support: - Seek emotional support from friends, family, or support groups. Living with diabetes can be emotionally challenging, and having a support system can provide comfort and understanding.

12. Stress Management: - Use stress-reduction techniques like meditation, deep breathing, or relaxation exercises to cope with the stress that may accompany managing a chronic condition.

13. Emotional Resilience: - Cultivate emotional resilience and a positive attitude. Focus on your achievements and the progress you make in managing your diabetes.

14. Adapting to Changes: - Be prepared to adapt to changes in your health and lifestyle as you age. This may include modifying your diet, exercise routine, and medication regimen to meet your evolving needs.

15. Self-Care: - Prioritize self-care and self-compassion. Taking care of yourself physically and emotionally is essential for managing diabetes and aging well.

16. Support System: - Lean on your support system and communicate openly about your diabetes management needs and challenges. Those close to you can provide encouragement and assistance.

17. Diabetes Education: - Consider enrolling in diabetes education programs that address the specific needs of older adults. These programs can provide practical strategies for managing your condition.

18. Independence: - Strive for independence while being aware of your limitations. Make any necessary adjustments to your living environment to enhance safety and convenience.

Coping with the challenges of aging with diabetes requires a holistic approach to your physical, emotional, and mental well-being. Remember that you are not alone in this journey, and there are resources and healthcare professionals available to support you in living a fulfilling and healthy life as you age with diabetes.

CHAPTER TWELVE
CONCLUSION

In conclusion, diabetes is a complex and chronic condition that affects people of all ages, but the challenges and considerations surrounding diabetes management can vary significantly for individuals over the age of 50. Understanding diabetes, its prevalence, risks, and the importance of diet, nutrition, and physical activity in managing the condition are all crucial components of effective diabetes management for older adults.

Managing diabetes at an older age also involves building a comprehensive care team that may include healthcare providers, diabetes educators, dietitians, and mental health professionals. Regular monitoring of blood sugar, medication management, and maintaining a support system are key elements in maintaining good health and emotional well-being while living with diabetes.

As individuals age with diabetes, they must pay particular attention to their heart health, cope with the emotional aspects of the condition, and adapt to the changes that come with aging. Engaging in a proactive and balanced approach to diabetes management is essential for maintaining a high quality of life while aging with diabetes.

Remember that you are not alone in your journey with diabetes. There are numerous resources, healthcare professionals, support groups, and technologies available to assist you in managing your condition effectively and leading a fulfilling life. By staying informed, seeking support, and staying committed to self-care, you can navigate the challenges of aging with diabetes and enjoy a healthy and rewarding life.

www.ingramcontent.com/pod-product-compliance
Lightning Source LLC
Chambersburg PA
CBHW050833260726
48660CB00006B/2211